# † SHIVA DICE †

Also by NJ Travis

† HOUSE OF PAIN †
(Vol. 1/Jasmine)

# † SHIVA DICE †

**(House of Pain, Vol. 2/Lotus)**

**NJ Travis**

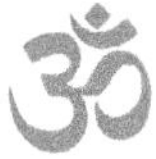

**LOTUS WELLBEING, INC. PUBLICATIONS**

LOTUS WELLBEING, INC. PUBLICATIONS

Shiva Dice (House of Pain, Volume 2)
NJ Travis



Cover Art: Vincent Stephens
Cover Design: NJ Travis, PYT, RYT-500
Copyediting: Jessica Winston, RYT

Web: www.lotuswellbeing.com

ISBN 978-0-61581-480-3 (paperback)



First Edition

For TJ and the Lost Boys

*"Only the deep study of the human heart, one of nature's most intricate labyrinths, can inspire the novelist whose work must show us man stripped bare...as he might become after his vices are corrected and he has been subjected to the commotions of passion." ~ The Marquis de Sade*

## Preface

Not having adequately disposed of my friends in the first volume of House of Pain, I'm no longer apologizing for abusing them with the corrective lessons necessary for enlightenment. Nor can I leave them in peace; we are still evolving spiritually. We have unfinished business: I with them and they with me.

†

While I was careful to explain the core concepts of Yoga, Tantra and Ayurveda in the first volume, Shiva Dice assumes that you now understand what I'm talking about. However with all kindness to the reader—I am not a sadist even on the literary level—this volume includes an appendix of the Sanskrit and yoga terms previously explained in House of Pain.

† May all Beings be Free †

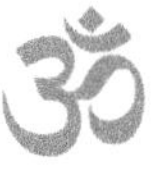

NJ Travis, PYT, RYT-500
Point Richmond, California
Bastille Day, July 14th, 2013

## † Acknowledgements †

Original cover art by Vincent Stephens **https://www.facebook.com/RamStar**

Hafiz quotations from “The Gift”, translations by Daniel Ladinsky

Sappho and Sanskrit mantra translations by NJ Travis

Botanical blends and medicinal properties are derived from the work of master alchemist and teacher, David Crow of Floracopeia, available at **http://bit.ly/YwBL83**

Much love to David Simon, M.D. co-founder of the Chopra Center for Wellbeing for sharing his love of botanical and alternative medicines.
**http://bit.ly/ZEJLL3**

Thank you to my colleague and friend, Jessica Winston, yoga and meditation teacher and marketing guru, for her thoughtful editing and encouragement.

Love to Steven Adler, the beautiful naked drummer boy—when he’s not dressed in leather and lace. (Guns ‘n Roses, Adler, “My Appetite for Destruction”)

OXO to Randy M. for rocking the world

# † SHIVA DICE †

# PROLOGUE

†

## BABY

Have I ever told you about the time I surfed the Point, just Roger and me, with a full police escort? It was shortly after the place had been over-run by drug dealers and was going straight to the dogs.

Murders on the beach, rapes, gang wars and heroin over-doses were becoming so common that only a handful of surfers bothered with it anymore. I thought twice about even looking at it, but Roger begged and I'm a fool for beggars, especially beautiful begging men.

Things are different now. The community fought back and cleaned the place up. It's safe for women and children again and it's not uncommon to see 70 surfers out on a beautiful Indian Summer swell like we had that day, just the two of us all alone at the peak.

I'll never forget Steven Mack, the mad man who took it upon himself to turn things around and almost died trying. S&M, nicknamed for his sheer contempt of pain and human suffering, is now the President and one of the founders of Sunrise Wellbeing, a private facility up on the top of the mountain for physical, mental and drug rehabilitation.

S&M was a notorious surfer, Tantric yoga teacher and the ringleader of the Point Guard, the self-styled 'guardian angels' of the beach. He was shot twice, point blank, right there on the beach by a couple of gang banger cartel kids, while he was strutting down the beach like a red-hot stripper on a summer day, right in front of his best friends.

A couple months later his motley crew of rehabilitated junkies, psychos and derelicts won the Point Guard team surf challenge and raised three-quarters of a million dollars for law enforcement and rehabilitation on a beautiful Sunday afternoon.

And that's what I wandered into, driving through a police barricade, right smack into the contest finals.

S&M personally invited me to stay while they polished off the competition, to have a go at the surf perfection when they were finished. A police officer valet parked my van and they kept the street shut down so we could quench our thirst for waves.

When we were done surfing, I thanked him and his team, the beautiful surf goddess Nicky with her young psychotic husband Kama Dave the God of Love, and wild Billy Lee who's now back on the professional tour after kicking heroin.

I met S&M's partner Officer Sean who helped found the Point Guard years ago to keep the kids safe, and his trainer and bodyguard Dr. Jain who spent eleven hours in surgery saving S&M's life when he was shot.

Then we followed them back up the mountain for a huge victory party where I met his brother Dr. Mack, his assistant yoga therapist Nat, his cute little personal chef Prince Albert and his two nurses, Sunny and his wife Brandy.

Crazy, all of them. Crazy as the day is long and the night is beautiful and I'll never forget them. It brings a smile to my face whenever I think of S&M still up there on the top of the world plotting to destroy all of humanity's pain and suffering, having taken the bodhisattva vow to bring enlightenment to the whole planet or to die trying.

## Part One: DARK AND TWISTED

***"The aim of practice is knowledge, dispassion, devotion, power and peace"*** ~ **Swami Satyananda**

# Part One: Dark and Twisted

†

NICK

It's hitting him at 2am every night now, occasionally a little earlier if he's having horror dreams. I can feel it coming like a distant train whistle. First I feel him sweating and then he's breathing hard. And suddenly he wakes up talking nonsense.

"No no no no," he wails and I have to rock him in my arms to calm him down.

"What's going on, baby?" I ask.

Tonight he says he's locked underground and can't find the way back up. His van is missing; someone took it. He's wandering around in a landscape that changes at every turn. And he's lost, hopelessly lost.

"Nah, it's just a bad dream, honey," I soothe him. "You don't have a van. You're safe in bed. Hold me. You're on top of the mountain. Everything is fine."

And then he buries his face in my neck and whispers, "I need my psychotics, Nick. Where are my psychotics?"

So I call Dr. Jain to give him another shot of lorazepam, because really what the boy needs is a sedative, an anti-psychotic. This one tends to work really well for him in the darkest hours before dawn when he seems to get strangled in the underworld.

In the morning he usually wakes up smiling with love and trust in his eyes. The thick wall that sometimes separates him from reality only surfaces when his guard is down. Usually he keeps it together and plays very nicely.

I knew he was mad when I married him; I knew he was twisted and afraid and had a dark unfathomable side to him, but it never stopped me for a minute. For the most part he is a gracious, loving and creative man.

The day before we were married Dr. Mack and Dr. Jain diagnosed him as a schizophrenic. His best friend and teacher, S&M, Steven Mack, vehemently disagrees. He says Dave's just going through an enlightenment phase.

Dave has a lot of the usual symptoms: delusions, hallucinations, suicidal tendencies, catatonic fits and confusion. But we couldn't get a thorough evaluation done by a psychiatrist because he has no family history that he'll share.

At first we thought the symptoms were the side effects of heroin withdrawal, but a little closer look at case studies made it clear that drug abuse is just another symptom of psychosis. Just about the only schizoid symptom he's missing is cigarette addiction. He's a yogi and a surfer and he hates to smoke.

"It's all just Maya," he laughed one day when we were getting flowers out of the lab. "None of this is fucking real. If you think that window is real, you're crazier than I am."

And when he smashes it with his fist and gets blood all over the lab countertop he proves his point. The window isn't there any more is it? Dr. Jain has gotten used to stitching him up by now and has even encouraged him to wear body builders' fingerless gloves to protect him.

The best bet is to just agree with him and keep him safe. Yes, baby, that window isn't really there any way, so there's no point in smashing it. Then he'll snort with joy and look pleased as punch that he's just conquered Maya by denying anything really exists.

I warm some milk with cinnamon, cardamom and vanilla and watch him calm down while we wait for Jain. When he sees the syringes he purrs, "oh my psychotics!" and within minutes of getting the hit, he drops into a kinder place.

David John is 21, but he's lost. S&M has filed for joint legal custody with me. Six years ago he found him living with a dog under the stairway to the beach, a half-naked 15 year old, eating garbage.

He took him home and fed him, but DJ was afraid to sleep in a room, so he let him sleep on the deck overlooking the ocean. Some mornings when he got up early to surf, DJ would be gone. Then walking down the beach to the Point, he'd spot him under the stairs talking to another stray.

Now we sleep upstairs in the drug-free house at Sunrise Wellbeing, where Dave is under six months court-ordered house arrest for narcotics rehabilitation in lieu of a prison sentence. Prison is guaranteed suicide for him. We figured that out even before we understood Dave is sick.

I ignored him for six years, thinking he was just a little annoying ADHD pest, but now we've been married for two months. I love him more than earth, water, fire, air and the space between us.

In the morning I hear him sigh and pull the pillow over his head without a word, instead of giving me his usual sweet good morning kiss. I try to pull the pillow off but he punches my arm away and moans, “No, no!”

I pull really hard and get the pillow but he puts his hands over his face and disappears into his own darkness.

“Baby?” I ask gently, “Aren’t you going to kiss me good morning?”

“Nicky, no,” he squirms shaking his head behind his open hands. “I need psychotics.”

“You had some at 2am,” I remind him. “You don’t need them in the morning. Just for the nightmares. You’re fine.”

“Nicky, no. I want them. Get them.”

I call Dr. Jain and explain the problem and he says no. He shouldn’t take any more. Just talk to him, okay? See if you can calm him down. Call me back in ten minutes.

“Jain said no, baby. He said to talk to me.”

He opens his eyes, glares at me in furor and grabs the phone to call his nurse. “Bran, I missed my psychotics last night. I need them now!” he hisses into the phone. Brandy can hear it in his voice. He’s frantic and shaken but she knows him well enough to know that’s he’s easily lying or just imagining things.

“Let me speak to Nicky, honey,” she says. He hangs up on her and starts to cry.

“Come on, sweetheart,” I purr. “Let me kiss you and make it better.”

And that just backfires on me.

“Don’t fucking look at me,” he screams. “Don’t fucking touch me. Shut up.”

He pushes my arms away and jumps out of bed naked and opens the window all the way.

“I’m leaving,” he announces and swings his leg over the second story window sill.

“Wait a second,” I warn. “That’s not going to kill you, baby Dave. It’s just going to break your legs and you won't be able to surf with us anymore."

He purses his lips and frowns.

"If you think for a minute that ground is real, you're crazier than I am," he laughs.

And then he hears Brandy call his name and he looks out the window and waves at her as she's coming down the path to the house.

"Oh, my psychotics," he purrs and climbs back into the bed. "She's here."

She runs up the stairs and comes in without knocking. I'm still a little shaken up as I'm struggling to close the window.

"We'll put a lock on that today," she promises. "Holy shit, Dave. Are you thinking of flying away or what?"

He gives her his innocent boy look like he hasn't got a clue what she's talking about. "Where are my psychotics, Bran?" he asks sweetly. "I don't see any needles."

"It's down in the lab, honey," she says. "I was in a hurry to see you first. Can you talk to me for a minute?"

"I might not, Bran. You promised. I want them."

"I think it's a good idea, Nicky," she says. "I'll tell Dr. Jain. I'll get some for him." She turns back to the door, but he stops her.

"I can talk to you first, Bran," he smirks. "A secret talk."

She sits on the edge of the bed and pets his hair and he leans over to whisper in her ear. He puts his fist up to his mouth and sucks on his knuckles while he's whispering.

"What?" she looks surprised. "Your what?"

"My narcotics," he says a little louder with his fist still in his mouth. "I want that one instead."

"Narcotics?" she raises her eyebrows. "You quit doing that months ago. You don't want that."

"Yes, I do. Dr. Mack will give me some morphine if I'm good. I've been very good but I have a headache now so I want some narcotics."

Brandy signals me by putting her hand around her wrist. I was thinking the same thing. I pull the restraining cuffs out of the bedside table and hand them to her. After all, she's his nurse. I'm just his prisoner. He'll listen to her.

"Sure, baby," she says. "Let's just play a little bit while we wait for Sunny to bring the morphine up."

His eyes light up and he laughs as she cuffs him to the bed headboard. He glares at me with his I-told-you-so smirk. He thinks he's running the show now.

"Lots of it, Bran," he prompts her.

She picks up the phone and dials S&M's number instead of Sunny's office and says sweetly, "Hello, Sunny. Dave would like a shot of morphine this morning. Would you bring it up? Lots of it, please. Okay. See you soon."

Then she turns back to Dave and says, "Now what game would you like to play today? Do you want to play with me or with Nicky?"

"I'm not speaking to her now, Bran. She tried to kiss me. I'd rather play with you. Pretend I'm a very sick boy and you're my nurse taking care of me. You can take my blood pressure if you like."

Brandy gets the blood pressure cuff and checks him while she purrs, "You poor sick boy. You need to rest now."

Just then the door swings open and S&M is standing there out of breath with his arms crossed.

"What the fuck, baby brother? Are you out of your mind trying to order narcotics when you're in rehab?"

"Yes, Nim," he laughs. "I'm a fucking lunatic. I'm crazy. Morphine is almost as nice as heroin if you can get lots of it. Heroin is seven times stronger than morphine."

"Nurse," he growls at his wife, "Get rid of the cuffs."

"No, I'm playing with her, Nim," he complains. "We're playing nurse."

"Honey, you're playing with *me* now. Get out of bed. You've been spending way too much time fucking and not enough time smashing things. It's enough to make anybody mentally unbalanced. Get your gloves on. Oh. And put some pants on while you're at it."

While Dave gets organized, I quietly explain to S&M that Dave was planning to jump out of the window naked when he thought he couldn't get any drugs. And just as soon as he thought they were on the way, he turned into Prince Fun 'n' Games Charming.

"I've got this Nicky," he promises. "I'll get him sorted out. Why don't you ladies take a little trip to the hardware store and get a padlock for the window?"

†

S&M

"Hey, Jain, I'm taking Dave out to play in the gym," I tell the doc on our way out. "The girls are going to the hardware store if you need anything."

"You okay, Dave?" he asks looking concerned. "I told him no more anti-psychotics this morning. Nick was supposed to call me back. I was just going to check on him."

"I'm stunning, Doc," Dave laughs. "I was going to fly out the window. Then Bran was getting me narcotics but now Nim wants to play with me."

He leans over and whispers in my ear, "Can I have some hardware too, Nim?"

"Depends on what kind of stuff."

"Rope could be a lot of fun," he sniffs.

"No rope. You'd probably try to hang yourself."

"No. Just to tie Nicky up and play prisoner."

"No rope."

"Um, how about a magnifying glass then? To look at stuff."

"We could get that if you promise not to try to burn the house down with it. Jain, can you ask the ladies to get him one and whatever kind of toys they think he might like. A puzzle might be good for him. Lots of pieces."

"Dice!"

"Okay, you're a cheap date, baby. Dice, too. And maybe some play money so we can gamble without losing our clothes. Let's go," I slap him on the back.

We walk out into the early morning sunshine; dew is glistening like broken glass on the lawn. Dave's got his jeans on and nothing else but a crystal pendant and sunglasses. I'm pretty much dressed the same except I'm wearing a silver necklace with a handcuff charm.

"What's it going to be then, Nim? Chest and arms?"

"Nah, no weight lifting today. We're playing something else."

I walk him over to the middle of the lawn where there's no equipment or furniture nearby and take his sunglasses off his face.

"Why?" he wonders as I walk back to the lawn sofa and put both our glasses in a safe place.

"We're going to play smash-up, honey," I say. "We're going to make a mess."

I put both my hands on his shoulders and step back at arm's length.

"What are the rules?" he asks.

"Probably only one. Don't kick me in the balls. Are you ready?"

He nods and grins so I have to wait until his smile fades before I hit him. I don't want to knock any of his pretty teeth out. And then I plant a nice punch on the left side of his face. I feel it connect and vibrate all the way down to my bare feet.

"What the fuck?" he cries. "You fucking belted me, Nim!"

His mouth is wide open in astonishment. It works even better than electroshock therapy.

"When was the last time I hit you?" I ask innocently.

"Never!"

"Yeah, that's what I thought. When was the last time you hit me?"

"Never. I don't know how to fight."

"Sure you do. You just never do it. But you put your fist through the medicine cabinet window a few times now so I'll bet you've got a pretty amazing sucker punch. Go ahead." I point to my chin.

He shakes his head and looks confused.

"You hit me!" he repeats astonished.

"Does it hurt?" I ask.

Then suddenly he bursts out laughing. "No! It doesn't hurt at all. It was just—surprising!"

"Come on then," I tease him. "It's really fun, especially if you're not mad and you're careful not to hurt each other. Don't hit below the belt. And try not to hit me in the eye. Game on!"

I snarl and slap myself in the face to demonstrate. His grin turns back on like the rising sun and he smacks me in the face so hard he knocks me off my feet. Not bad for a little guy.

"Does it hurt, Nim?" He looks a little worried.

"Not at all," I laugh. "It's just fucking amazing. All that window smashing is paying off. But that's the last free throw you get, buddy."

I jump up and give him a body shot and then block his next punch. I never lose but I don't want him to get frustrated with it, so I show him how to use both hands, how to block, hook, cross, uppercut and speed jab. We're just sparring for an hour or so, no rules, no agenda, just nice and easy.

When he starts working with his left fist, he gets some nice hits because that hand has never been broken. Then I show him how to land a bolo punch and put my guard down so he can get the hang of it. He almost takes the nose off my face with his left fist.

He roars with laughter. "Fuck. You have blood on you, Nim!"

"You little blood sucking pervert," I hiss as I hammer him in the solar plexus and follow it with an upper cut. He's laughing so hard he bites his lip when I hit him. And then he licks it, tastes the blood and snorts with joy.

"Done," I declare. "Tie! Usually in sparring we stop at first blood, but I let you take that shot. And you know I never fucking lose, so it has to be a tie. Even though you technically won."

"Unreal, I won! And it's only my first fight."

"You're dead if you tell anyone," I growl. "I let you hit me."

Nicky and Brandy are walking up the path with a couple bags and he yells when he sees them.

"I fucking won! My first fight! I cannot lose!"

I just shake my head. It's good to see him so happy.

Brandy and Nicky are frowning in disbelief. I wipe the blood off my mouth with the back of my hand and give them my best drop-dead lady killer smile and explain.

"Too much fucking and not enough fighting will drive any man nuts. You've got to take it easy on the poor boy, Nicky. You're driving him crazy with all that Tantric sex."

Nicky doesn't say a word. She pulls some tissue out of her pocket and wipes the blood off his lip. She gives him a peck on the cheek, but he grabs her and plants a huge French kiss on her mouth so she can taste his beautiful blood.

"Are you feeling better, honey?" Brandy asks him. In spite of the cut on his lip, he looks like he just won the lottery. He grins and licks his lips. Then he gives her a huge kiss as well.

"Hang on, Dave," I protest. "You can't be kissing my wife like that."

"Just one, Nim," he laughs. "But no sex."

Nicky takes another tissue and cleans my face and then she gives me one of those straight-laced respectful kisses that she's been giving me for six years. No tongue or even a trace of heat, she kisses me just like she's my sister.

"You're such a beautiful loser, S&M," she teases.

"Get lost, Nicky," I sneer. "Have Jain take care of the window and we'll be in to check out the toys pretty soon."

"Okay, Dave," I point to the grass, "have a seat. I want to talk to you, buddy."

He's in the best mood I've seen since he got married, so I reckon we might throw some light into the darkness. He sits on the soft grass in lotus position, perfectly at ease with a soft Buddha smile on his split lip and I sit down facing him.

"Tell me. Before you were living on the street. Where was your home? Where were you from?"

His face turns dark and the smile disappears like a cloud swallowing the sun.

"I am not from anywhere," he says flatly. "I don't have a home."

"Come on. I want to help you. We can get rid of some of the nightmares if you open up a little. I know you trust me. Just talk to me."

"No. I won't go back."

"And you never have to. We've got you, baby. Nick and I have legal guardianship and you're 21, an adult now anyway. It's okay to talk about these things. I know a lot of bad things can happen to street kids. Drugs and rape and abduction and disease – "

He unfolds his legs and gets to his feet. "Fuck off, Steven," he says. "Don't fucking talk to me."

I grab his arm and pull him back down and pin him to the grass in a submission lock.

"Don't ever call me fucking Steven again," I threaten. "It sounds like you're spitting at me the way you said it."

He frowns and shuts his eyes to disappear, but I won't let him go.

"Kama Dave," I purr sweetly. "How old were you when you ran away from home?"

"How do you know?" he opens his eyes and stares at me in wonder. "I didn't tell you that."

"It's the same old story, honey. It's the usual way kids get out on their own too soon. My parents died when I was 13 but my brother was old enough to get custody and he took care of me—when he was looking anyway. I got away with murder but I always had someone to clean up my mess."

He sneers, "I lost my parents when I was 13, too. But I just divorced them. I don't even remember where they live. They were just fucked up people. They couldn't be my real parents. Sometimes babies get mixed up in the hospital. I don't have real parents."

"They hurt you?"

"Nothing hurts me, Nim. You know that. Nothing can even touch me. It's just an illusion."

I let go of him and ask him to sit nicely again and he goes back into lotus position and breathes. He pulls a little bottle of jasmine oil out of his pocket and sniffs it first through his left nostril then through the right.

"Good boy," I say. "Bad stuff happens. It's not your fault. Bad stuff happened so you ran away, right?"

He nods watching his toes on his lap.

"No. Look me in the eye. You trust me. Then worse bad stuff happened after you ran away, right?"

He rips into me with a dirty glare and his fists ball up, but he nods his head.

"Right."

"And you don't want to talk about it. I get it. Will you talk to Nat? Will you do some therapy with her?"

He shakes his head no.

"Okay, then. Don't get mad at me, but let me guess. I know it freaks you out to get locked up. Maybe your fake parents locked you up. And when you ran away maybe someone offered to help you, to keep you safe. And then they hurt you instead. Maybe someone gave you drugs or drinks and locked you up and did things to you. And you had no clue what was happening to you. Just a wild guess but you know what? It happens *all the time* to runaway kids!"

He starts to cry but snorts it back and begs, "Don't do this to me, Nim. Please don't. This hurts."

"Nah," I say. "This helps, but that's enough now. Come on."

I get up and help him to his feet.

"I think we need some lunch. And some bourbon. The ladies have bought some nice things for you."

"For me?"

"Yeah. Are you still mad at Nicky?"

"No, Nim. I love Nicky. I'm never mad at Nicky."

"Good. Tomorrow I'll teach you how to do a proper strip tease. She's going to love it. It's going to make her scream."

†

DJ

Now I know how to fuck and I know how to fight. Tomorrow I'm going to learn how to strip. It just keeps getting better. Before we go in the house, I ask Nim something that's been worrying me since they filed the court papers to get custody.

"If you and Nicky are my guardians then you're like my new father and mother. But Nicky is my wife. So does that make me a mother fucker?"

Nim howls like a mad dog.

"Nah. Too funny! No, we didn't adopt you. It's just that if you ever have trouble taking care of yourself, we've got you. Like when my brother had custody over me, he wasn't my father, he was my guardian."

"Too bad. You would make a good father."

"There are probably 100 or so kids out there who would disagree with you, but never mind. If you want me to be your father, I could adopt you. Then Brandy would be your mother and if you fucked with *her*, then yes, you would be one very dead mother fucker. And you wouldn't be kissing your mother like you kissed her today either."

"Cool," I say. "Very cool. I was worried about it. I think I get it now."

I almost forget about it when we go in the kitchen because Prince has made piles of cheese sandwiches and a mountain of potato egg salad. Nim pours us some bourbon and we sit at the boardroom table with Nicky, Brandy and Prince. Prince can't have any drinks because he's only 18. He only gets lemonade and the ladies like that too.

"Um, Nicky?" Nim wonders. "What would you think if I adopted your husband? Is that too weird?"

She crunches her nose and tilts her head as if to let the thought run in one ear and out the other.

"That's pretty kinky, baby. You'd be my father-in-law and you're younger then me. Go for it."

Brandy's gears start turning too and she stares at me.

"Baby Dave, you're like my little brother. But I could be your mother, too. No problem."

Then Nicky starts laughing. "S&M, if we adopt one of your bastards he'd be your son and your grandson, too. That's just twisted. Oh my, Brandy! Forget I ever said that. Where are my manners? It's only speculation. There's absolutely no proof he has any kids." She chokes on the potato salad laughing.

"Well, it's a thought," he says. "We might need a computer to sort it all out. I'll think about it."

Nim pours us more bourbon with three drops of orange bitters and cherries and Brandy pulls out a shopping bag stuffed with—stuff. A monstrous puzzle of a water lily pond painting, deadly difficult with little Monet paint points. A sweet magnifying glass map reader in the shape of a ship's steering wheel with eight brass compass pointers around it. A dozen green and red dice and a stack of play money, $10,000 worth. A pair of toy handcuffs that don't need a key. A nice new razor.

I think I should try to jump out of the window more often; they're spoiling me so rotten. I wonder what else I can ask for now whilst I'm being so pampered. I put my dirty feet up on the table and make a sad face at Brandy.

"Mom? Can I have a foot massage please with sugar on it?" Now my nurse is my mother too. Even if they don't adopt me, I've already decided to adopt them. Nim and Brandy are very good parents for me. I'm pretending they're my real parents who got their baby mixed up and lost in the hospital.

Nim sneers at me. "Don't press your luck, son. I know how your twisted little mind works."

But Brandy gets a washcloth and oil and cleans my bare feet and carefully rubs the sandalwood and jasmine into my soles and around my toes. Brandy massages like a nurse, very caring and thorough. Nicky massages like a Tantric sex freak. I can't have her doing that to me in public. I would be moaning and groaning all over the place.

"Prince," Nim says to his personal chef, "how old were you when you ran away from home?"

"Eleven," he says.

"Pretty scary?"

"Hell yes," Prince swears. He never uses dirty words, so I'm shocked.

"Did you ever have bad stuff happen to you on the street?"

"Things I wouldn't talk about at the table. Pretty terrible things. Which was why I started dealing dope, to get off the street. I was dealing when I was 12. It was the smartest thing I ever did. That is, before you hired me."

"Why did you run away?" he continues.

"My parents were brutal. They beat each other and then they beat me. They locked me out of the house all the time and I had to sleep in the yard with the dog."

"I slept with a dog, too!" I laugh. "I had a really good beach dog for a while."

"Okay thanks, Prince," Nim says. "No need to talk about it at the table. I was just wondering if you could talk to Dave about it sometime. I'll bet you guys could be pretty good friends."

"Sure thing, any time," he nods. "Maybe he could explain to me why he is so psycho."

"Maybe he could. You guys could help each other out, teach each other stuff."

"I know how to fight now, Prince," I brag. "I beat Nim up and bloodied his nose. It was killer."

"I don't think I want to learn how to fight, Dave. I'd rather cook. I've been hit enough already." He looks at Nim and smiles a fake smile. "I don't much like it. But maybe he could explain to me how he married—her. She's—uh, awesome."

He stares at Nicky and she blushes. "You're pretty sweet yourself, sugar." She winks at him.

"Nicky! You aren't allowed to fool around with him," I command her. "No kissing. No winking. No tucking him in bed. You're my prisoner. Don't forget who you belong to or I'll—jump out of the window and kill myself."

"Please don't hurt yourself, baby Dave," she purrs. "A wink is just a private joke. It can mean you're not serious, you're just kidding."

And then she winks at me and I don't know if that's a joke or if maybe she's not serious about winking not being serious. I'm so confused that I want to cry but I have a big pile of gifts and a foot massage and my brand new parents and bourbon, so I don't cry. Instead I wink at Prince and his jaw drops out of shock.

†

## PRINCE ALBERT

I'm not too excited about making friends with the psycho crybaby, but there's no one else near my age here. Everyone else is at least 10 years older and I can't trust anyone over 21. I sure don't trust *her*, because she's kissed me and winked at me and she's already married. And she's S&M's girl friend, too. How does that even happen?

After lunch I clean up the kitchen and put some stock on to simmer for dinner later and then kick back in my room to read. I've got it made here. I'm not under house arrest like Dave so I can borrow the car to go shopping or whatever I want. S&M is paying me a healthy salary and I've got no expenses in the world so I'm getting a fat little bank account.

S&M felt really bad about beating me up for selling dope and robbing me, but he's more than made up for it with a pile of awesome cookbooks. I spent a lot of time studying when I was too messed up to get up and cook. I've got The Complete Thomas Keller box set, Jacque Pépin's Fast Food My Way and an Ayurvedic one, Heaven's Banquet. I've got a lot more but I can rock the house with those three.

We haven't got TV or Internet in our house but I've got an MP3 player and Dr. Mack lets me download music and order books from the office computer. So I've got some screaming bad music in my room I can crank up over the headphones. I don't even know if Dave knocks on the door because I'm listening to Five Finger Death Punch so loud my ears are imploding.

But the door opens and I can see his lips move. I turn the music off and stare at him. He really makes me nervous. He's got a girl's necklace on, a busted lip and he doesn't own a shirt or shoes. You can't even work in a professional kitchen if you don't have a shirt and shoes.

"What are you reading?" he asks.

I show him the skull on the front. The book is 'My Appetite for Destruction' by Steven Adler.

"It's a true story about an 11 year old kid who got thrown out on the streets by his parents," I tell him. "He became one of the biggest rock star junkies of all time. He makes you look like an altar boy, Dave. I was smart to be a dope dealer instead of a junkie."

"Oh." He says. "Much sex in it?"

"Nothing but sex. It's very, very bad behavior. There's a lot of Q's and V's and coke and heroin and whiskey, but apparently no methamphetamine in it. You might like it. You can read it when I'm done."

"Yeah, I'd love to read it. But I don't know what Q's and V's are," he says and I laugh at him.

"You really don't know much about dope for a junkie. That's pretty funny. Q's and V's are Qualudes and Valium. Terrible stuff. I wouldn't even sell it. It's for perverts. They knock you unconscious and you don't even know what's happening. It's not a lot of fun."

"Oh. Do you want to play dice?" he quickly changes the subject. "I've only got play money but I can loan you $5,000 to start the game."

"I don't know how to play."

"That's even better. I know all the rules and the provisions you can cheat with. Nim taught us how and the whole house loves to play, so you should learn."

Why not? I think. He says it'll be easier to play on the floor and I really don't want him to sit on my bed even for a second so we get down on the floor. I get the green set and $5,000 and he starts showing me the rules. It's pretty easy. The Shiva Dice game only uses two dice and it's simple to play but the rules are twisted. Then Liar's Dice uses five dice and 4/24 uses all six.

I win $1,000 off him and he says it's just 'beginners luck'.

"Does the house play for real money ever?" I'm excited. I can get in on some house action. I'm into the money.

"Nah, we were playing for clothing, strip dice. Apparently that caused some problems for Dr. Jain so Nim got the play money today. The guys don't want to play for clothing if the ladies aren't in the game."

Okay, let me just come right out with it and ask him.

"How'd you get the babe? How did you do that? Do you have a lot of money or what?"

"I haven't got *any* money. I've only just now got this play money. I wouldn't know what to do with the real stuff. But I just waited and waited for her. Nim told her I had a warranty. I got some nice love oils and sex lessons from Nat. But first you have to learn your wiring, and understand the koshas and chakras, the big picture. That's why you do yoga.

"The most important thing I learned about sex is don't do it until they beg you. But you might get beaten up anyway. Be polite but wait until they start crying. Nim said not to look at them or talk to them or touch them. That's very smart because then they have to beg."

"Oh." It's my turn to be stupid. I don't know what he's talking about.

"She asked me to marry her 33 times. I wanted her to ask 99 times, but—"

"But what?"

"I fucking caved in," he snorts. "You're too young still. You should wait. If you just want a lesson, Sage will do it but Nim says she's dangerous. He can make a list of girls for you."

"What about Nat?" I ask.

"Nope. She's getting married to Dr. Jain. He'll punch you. He kicked my ass. What you want to do if you're serious is get a centerfold in the Sunday paper. Then you get 48 marriage proposals and hundreds of love letters. I can give you some of mine if you want. You can write back and say 'Sorry, Kama Dave is married now but Prince Albert is available.' And then you can send them a nice centerfold picture."

"That's a pretty good idea. I'll write to them."

"Ask Nim and he'll sort through the mail for you and give you a short list."

"Why do you call him Nim?" I wonder.

"It's short for S&M. But nobody else can call him that but me. Nobody else would know so don't even try to do it. Everyone else has to call him Sim. And don't ever call him fucking Steven or he'll hammer you. Only the staff can call him that because it's his legal name."

"Q's," I tell him, diving straight into the dirt that S&M asked me to talk to him about. "That's the terrible stuff I'm supposed to tell you. They take you home and give you Q's and the next thing you know you're fucked and you're lying in the street. But you don't know how it happened. I figured it out pretty quick but it wasn't nice.

"If a woman took you home, she would clean you up and feed you but never rape you. But don't get in the car with a strange guy because it always ends up with Q's and nothing even to eat, even if they seem nice. Especially if they seem nice."

He stares at me and his face goes white.

"You owe me $5,000," he finally says. "I've got to go."

"Didn't that ever happen to you?" I ask. "I'm not afraid to talk about it. I didn't agree so it doesn't count as sex. I'm still a virgin. I don't remember what happened. I got hurt a few times before I figured it out."

"Not like that it didn't," he mumbles. "I got fucking locked up and didn't even get the Q's, so I remember everything they did. But you're right. Don't get in the car even if they seem nice. The police make you get in the car and they'll lock you up and hit you if you cry, but it's never anything worse than some smacks. These psychos locked me in the closet and fucked me over for a week. I was 13. Then they found another boy and threw me out because I was screaming too much. It really helps to cry if it's psychos."

"Is that how you got so psychotic?" I wonder. "Did you catch it from them?"

"I don't know. It wasn't Disneyland," he shakes his head. "But there's a lot more than that. The whole world is making me nervous. Don't you ever wish it would stop spinning just for a little bit and stop making all those Om noises? It gets a little intense sometimes."

He looks at me for answers but I haven't got a clue what he's talking about. I'm counting out his $5,000 so he can take a nap before dinner when there's a knock on the door. It's S&M checking on us. He smiles when he sees the dice and the money.

"What are you guys talking about?" he wonders.

"Money," we both say at the same time.

And then I add, “I’m explaining investment banking to him because he never had any real money before.”

“Right,” S&M says. “Sex. I figured as much. Do you want to talk to me about it?

“No, thank you,” we both say in unison.

“Nim? Dad,” Dave commands like he’s in charge of the place, “Give Prince some of my centerfold mail so he can write back to them and say he’s available instead of me. Find some nice ones for him. He’s just a virgin if you don’t count abductions and cock sucking perverts.”

S&M shows us all his teeth and throws his head back to inspect the ceiling.

“Oh brother,” he laughs. “I’m not into reading your love letters, Dave. But I can give a stack of them to Nicky to review for him.”

“Cool,” I say. “I want to see their pictures. I’ve got money now. I’ve got freedom. They’ll love me.”

†

S&M

Prince is working in the kitchen when I come out of the lab. Nat’s just finished knocking me into yoga nidra conscious dreaming for an hour after abhyanga with hot sandalwood oil. I’m feeling translucent, impeccable, inviolable. I feel like Shiva Nataraj dancing in order to make the world rock. Hell no. I don’t just feel like Shiva, I am Shiva.

“What’s for dinner?” I poke my nose over the stove to see where all the exotic smells are coming from.

“Pretty simple tonight,” he says. “It’s just creamy polenta with manchego cheese but it’s going to be made with this homemade veggie broth and toasted spice. Nat gave me the yogi spice recipe. Toasted coriander and fennel seeds, red, white and black peppercorns and pink Himalayan mineral salt. It's brilliant. Then it's rack of lamb rubbed with the same spice mix, roasted cherry vinegar sauce and Greek salad."

"Yum," I approve. "Do you need a raise?"

"Sure. I'm all about the money. I need a new cell phone to call all those babes."

"Yeah, you and my buddy Billy both, all about the money. How did you get along with Dave?"

"He's not as scary as I thought, now that I understand why he's so psycho. I didn't know that was catchy. I just hope I don't get it."

"Uh, what? No it's not catchy. Hey, just so you know, part of what's going on with Dave is delusions. He's not always telling you the truth although he thinks he is. I mean he's not lying, but sometimes he can drop the connection.

"In yoga, we call it Vairagia, dispassion, non-attachment to the world. I don't know if he's crazy or enlightened. It could be a little of both with him. He studied yoga with me for years and dispassion is actually one of the supreme goals of yoga. He can meditate like a son of a bitch right into catatonic bliss."

"Oh yeah?" I wonder. "Dave told me the reason you do yoga is to figure out the big picture for sex."

"Absolutely not. He's just miscommunicating. Sex is a side affect. He knows better. The reason you do yoga is to achieve the divine qualities of knowledge, dispassion, devotion, power and peace. Money can't buy that.

"I know you don't want to talk about sex but there's nothing like it if you've got those qualities. You'll never screw it up. So I'd agree with him on one thing. Sex is not the goal of yoga, but if that's the impetus that starts you on the path, it's as good as any."

I fucking make him nervous. I can feel his pranic energy rolling off him like sheets of glass, splintered and cracked, so I take a few steps back and sit in one of the kitchen chairs. I hate to see him learn everything from delusional Dave because I can tell he's got a few of his own wires crossed already.

"Can I tell you something in confidence?" I ask, knowing that's an oxymoron to ask of a teenager.

He nods and makes a little rare eye contact so I trust he's with me.

"When I was your age, I probably fathered a hundred kids. We're still counting. I didn't give a shit then and it will take the rest of my life to clean up all that bad karma.

"Don't be in such a rush. There's no such thing as casual sex. No such thing as casual anything. Everything you do has karmic consequences embedded in your soul permanently. Not to scare you, buddy, but sex involves every cell of your body, every beat of your heart."

"What time do you want dinner on?" he asks, quickly changing the subject.

"Six is fine. Can I taste the broth?"

He's done a beautiful job of it. There's really only one way you can fuck up vegetables and that's by beating them to death. They're alive. They need to be coaxed and spiced and dressed.

"Yeah, man," I purr. "It's under-salted but you know what you're doing. You did that on purpose, right?"

"Right. You can always add more salt at the end, but if you have too much, you can never take it away."

"My point exactly," I smile. "I can never take back the pain I caused. Less is nicer."

"So what are you saying?" he asks. I feel like he's hearing me for the first time.

"I'm just saying write a hundred letters to one girl instead of writing to a hundred girls."

†

DJ

I have a deep nourishing nap and dream my sparkling water dreams again. The water dreams are the best, soft and safe underneath the ocean, not like the dark snaring earth underground. When I open my eyes Nicky is sitting by the window watching me, but the window is locked. I don't like that. I want to smash the window, but I've promised Nim not to hurt the house anymore. Instead I make a face at her and bite on my fat lip.

She laughs. "You let him hit you! I thought you didn't want to be hit, baby."

"*You* don't have permission to hit me," I frown. "That was just sparring with Nim, consensual hitting. I wouldn't ever hit you so we just can't do it."

She stares a little deeper and tips her head to the side, trying to see if she can look at me from another angle to see inside my head.

"Oh, that's too bad, baby," she purrs. "I could turn you into whipped cream if you let me. It wouldn't be bloody lips or noses, just a little bit of surprising."

She gets up and comes over to the bed and sits next to me, putting her hand in my hair, pulling my hair hard enough to sting me, pulling my head back while she kisses my mouth. Her tongue is warm and sweet and she's right. The hair pulling is a little surprising and I feel hot all of a sudden.

"S&M likes to play a little bit rough," she whispers, "but I never kiss him like that. This is only for you, honey. You looked so cute sleeping there with your cut lip, I started thinking about some roughhouse games and how sweet it would be if we could get all mixed up like whipping cream. A little kissing, a little biting, a little belt."

My face is starting to burn and I'm embarrassed, but she's asking me very nicely. I ask her to unlock the window to see if she'll obey me. She unlocks the padlock, puts it on the sill and opens the window a little bit, just enough for me to cool off.

"I don't know how to do it, Nicky," I explain. "I only just learned Tantric sex."

"Sure you do, baby. It's just a little connection between your body and your mind. It's mostly in your mind. Why are you blushing like that if it hasn't already gotten into your mind? Let me teach you."

And then she whispers in my ear, please with sugar, honey, cherry jam and whipped cream. *Please!* She takes my hand and tugs on me and hands me my jeans.

"With clothes," she instructs.

Just as soon as I get my jeans on she starts fussing around in the dresser and pulls out a little belt, nothing too scary looking, and threads it through my belt loops. I never wear one. And just as soon as she gets it fastened around my hips, she starts unfastening it again slowly and playing with the buckle and the button on my jeans and the zipper, like she's not sure if I should be dressed or not.

She puts her arms around me, one in my hair and the other stroking my naked back. She's purring like a big cat and biting my lip and my neck and my heart starts pounding. She's right again. My mind is going crazy just wondering and waiting for the surprise. I feel the heat rising from my toes to the tips of my ears and my head is spinning.

And then she pulls the chair over and takes both of my hands and puts them on the back of it.

"You don't like to be locked up, baby. So just hold on nicely and don't let go."

She stands behind me and holds me tight like we're two spoons in the drawer and pulls the belt all the way off me slowly. I hear her slap her hand gently with it and then I feel her hand running across the skin of my back and there's a loud crack. The sting disappears as fast as it comes and all of the sensations go straight to my cock.

She kisses my shoulder and nibbles on my skin and purrs some more. "Nice?" she asks and I don't understand how a belt could be nice, but I beg her to do it again. I can feel smoke coming out of my ears.

She walks around me and points to my hands and says, "Don't let go, please. I just want to look at you."

Then I get one hard kiss that hurts my mouth and she says, "You are the sweetest man on the planet, Kama Dave. I love you more than air, more than water." And she walks back around and belts me a lot harder and pulls my head back by my hair.

She puts her hand on my cock and laughs, "That worked pretty nicely didn't it? Is that enough for you, baby?" she whispers.

"One more please." I don't know why I beg for it but it just can't be over yet. I feel too hot to stop.

She laughs and gives me another hard smack across my back and then sits down in the little chair facing me looking up in my eyes. Right now I love her more than ever. I feel the river flooding all of the space between us. She kisses my hands and licks my belly and puts her tongue right inside my navel. She takes my cock out and pets me with both hands and I'm ready to dive straight into bed with her to play marriage.

But then she does something horribly bad that shocks me and worries me very much. She gets down on her knees and puts it in her mouth and I don't know what to do. I know that's very perverted and not to be done except by cock suckers and abductors so I yell for her to stop but all the things I say come out like a dog howling in the dark. I pull her hair to make her stop but then I end up just pushing her head down harder on me and helping her destroy me completely.

In less than a minute I'm down on my knees on the floor half in and half out of my jeans, looking straight into the snake green eyes of Kali as she's trying to kiss me again. I push her away and scream, Stop it. Fucking stop it.

I'm not a poor sick boy anymore. Now I'm just a fucking sick pervert married to a cocksucker. How does that even happen to a man in less than a minute? I just stare at her in shock and pull my jeans back on and get the fuck out of there.

†

## BRANDY

I promised Prince I'd bring some fresh herbs over for our dinner, so I'm trimming some long sprigs of thyme, sage and rosemary from the garden on the deck when I hear pounding at the front door of the pool house. When I open it there's Dave in his jeans looking horribly agitated and distraught.

"What's up, honey?" I coax. "You were so happy at lunch. Did you miss me?"

He just looks at his feet so I take his arm and lead him out back to sit on the futon on the deck. It's one of his favorite places and he relaxes slightly and looks around at the treetops and then lets out a horrid pathetic sigh.

"Are you looking for drugs again?" I ask. I put my arm around his shoulders and hug him. "You're not supposed to be alone. Do you want tea? Bourbon? What can I do?"

"Tea with bourbon," he says. "Lots of it. But no more drugs. I need to think about this."

"Okay, you just breathe while I get a drink for you. Do yogi breathing with your oil."

When I come back, he's obediently sniffing on his jasmine oil and staring into space.

"Thanks, Mom," he says absently. He takes a big drink and says, "I need to get a divorce. Can I sleep here for now?"

The phone starts ringing in the bedroom so I leave him alone for a minute. It's Nicky, just as upset as Dave.

"Is he there?" she's crying. "He just ran away. We were having sex and he totally freaked on me, Brandy. Is he okay? Does he need his drugs?"

"Give me some time, Nicky. Let me talk to him. I don't know what's going on yet. Give me a few minutes and I'll get back to you. Stay by the phone."

Before I go back out, I call the office to see if Sim can come over and give me some help.

"He's off the rails again, honey," I warn him. "Drugs won't fix this." I know Sim's at the end of his tether and doesn't want to have DJ sleeping with us again. He groans and hangs up, but I know he's on his way. And then I sit back down with Dave.

"Why would you need a divorce, baby? You love Nicky. That's not nice to say."

"I love her, Brandy, but she's very, very bad. Irreconcilable divorce," he moans.

"What happened? She's worried about you, honey. She said you freaked out."

"She's the one who freaked out," he hisses. "How would I know? Why didn't someone warn me? She's a fucking pervert!"

Sim walks in the door just in time to catch that. "Hmmm, who's the pervert now?" he laughs. "I thought you took the cake, Kamadev."

"No, this is serious," he moans. "She's sick, Nim. I need a divorce."

"My girl Nicky is sick? She's a lot less twisted than you, honey. But tell me all about it, son. I need to hear a lot more about sickness to get my mind off your problems. What did she do? Hit you?"

Dave puts his head down and then looks up defiantly. "I liked that part, Nim," he groans. "She made me into whipped cream. She did it very nice and sweet."

Sim smiles at that and says, "Oh, good boy!" and picks up the phone and calls her. "Okay, Nicky, I told you to go easy on the poor kid with all that Tantric sex. I mean it, I told you this morning. What the fuck have you done, girl friend?"

He listens for a minute and says, "No that's fine, Nick, that's cool, that's consensual. No harm done. And then? Oh! First time? No, you've just got to slow it down, honey. He may be the God of Love but he's got the sexual maturity of a 13 year old. He doesn't know what straight is. You almost got a divorce, you beautiful little cocksucker."

Dave's mouth drops when he hears that word and he stares at Sim. And Sim just smiles at me and says, "Who's going to explain this to him, Mom? You or me?"

"Explain what?" I ask.

"I told her to go easy on him so she did about the nicest thing she could think of, a pure and simple blow job. And he's probably only ever heard about sexual predators doing that so he thinks it's wrong. So do you want to explain, Mom?"

"Oh!" I start giggling and Dave turns red with anger. "No, I'm not laughing at you, baby. What she did is just a very special married treat. There's nothing wrong with that. She's not a pervert; she was giving you a very nice present."

"How would I know?" he whines.

"Ask me, honey," Sim says kindly. "Ask me anything if you get confused. Nicky is a kinky girl but she's not a predator. She loves you. I picked her just for you. I'd understand it if she wanted a divorce because you're so psychotic, but you'd be mad to leave her. Hell, you are mad, aren't you? You'll never find a nicer girl. Brandy, can you get him another drink? Me, too."

Dave is staring at Sim, a little excited now. "Do you mean it's okay? You would do that?"

"Fuck yes, buddy," he says. "It's better than okay. There's nothing wrong with love. And there's nothing you can do wrong with sex if you do it with love and devotion. Was it nice?"

"It was too fast, Nim. It was too surprising."

"You need to try it again, but ask her to slow it down a little. Trust me. It'll put you to sleep like a baby without any drugs.

"What do I do now?" he wonders shaking his head.

"Well, for one thing, you hurt her feelings. You probably should go home for dinner and let her know you're sorry. The rest is a piece of cake.

You're either going to figure it out or take anti-psychotics the rest of your life. What do you think?"

†

DJ

Bran cut a white rose for me to bring home as an apology. The rose has sharp spiked thorns all along the stem and I play with the little prickly points as we walk back to the Fire House for dinner, me with Nim and Brandy.

No one talks so I just think about what I have to say. Then I think how their silence speaks so much clearer than their words. They're not trying to tell me what to do. They trust me to figure it out. All of a sudden I understand that I don't have to say anything to her at all.

Before we go through the kitchen door, Brandy picks some jasmine for my hair and kisses me like a mother. When we walk in, everyone is already sitting around the table in the boardroom waiting for us. Prince starts bringing out platters of food family style from the kitchen. Nim follows him in first and sits down next to Nicky, then Brandy walks around the table and I follow her.

When I walk behind Nicky I pull her hair as I go past so she knows I'm here, and so she'll know that I remember the roughhouse games. I put the rose down by her plate, but I don't say a word. I have a nice plan. I pull out the chair across from Nim for Brandy to sit down, politely like a perfectly obedient boy. And then I stand behind the empty chair next to her, across from Nicky.

But I don't sit down. I just wait and stare at Nicky until she looks up at me with sad green eyes. Then I hold both my hands out, grip the back of my chair and stand there holding on nicely, smiling the best lady killer smile I've copied from Nim.

I hold the chair so she could belt me or kiss me or bite me or pull my hair if she wanted. I watch the corners of her mouth curl up like the soft petals of the rose and I wish the rose I gave her were pink like her mouth.

I'm breathing hard already but I cool it down and wait. She gives me a little wink and taps the top of the table with her fingernail once for me to sit down. Nim is staring at us and he laughs hard and nods his head in approval.

Then they start passing around the beautiful dishes. I pile a mountain of polenta on my plate, then a few lamb chops and I spoon roasted cherry sauce over the top of everything.

I'm so hungry I don't know what to do with myself. I'm hungry in my body, mind and soul. When I look up she's giving me a shy look and I smile at her again. I'm ready for a hot oil bath and bed instead of this food.

I want to touch every inch of her and rub the flower oils into her skin, the saffron and rose. I try to see if I can touch her feet with mine under the table but the boardroom table is too big and wide, so I just keep leering at her.

She looks at my giant plate of food and asks, "Is that enough for you, baby?" It's the same words she used during the belt game and I laugh and shake my head no. "Would you like some more?" she teases and I'm grinning yes like the Cheshire cat.

Nim and Brandy are both laughing at us now, but no one else at the table notices the games. Brandy puts her hand on my shoulder and whispers, "Eat your dinner, honey. Or you don't get any whipped cream for dessert."

I pick up a piece of lamb with my fingers and bite into it and the spices pop in my mouth with peppery sweetness, hot and cool at the same time. I'm digging ravenously into it now, nearly drowning in the cherry sauce.

I can taste the softness in the sharp cheese, the silkiness in the bite of the cornmeal, sweet sugar in the tart cherry, the pleasure inside of pain. I feel Brandy's hand on my leg and she whispers, slow it down, take your time, hungry boy.

But I can eat the whole world now because I finally know. And what I know fills my whole body with warm green light that reaches all the way across the table and makes Nicky blush deliciously. I'm fucking her with my heart without even touching her, with my eyes, in public, without anyone else in the room knowing.

I remember she was sitting on the bedroom chair and I loved her more than ever and I go right back there, before I was surprised, when I could taste how much she really loved me.

She can see it in my eyes, that I'm not sick any more. I'm not her broken boy toy. The game has opened the river again and the water is pouring through my mind through the channel of my heart and filling up the reservoir of my soul. I'm home again. I can taste her. She tastes like pure love.

†

## NICK

He eats like a pig, but he never takes his eyes off me. For the first time, he looks like a stranger, like I've never seen him before. The little lost boy has disappeared and he looks as serious as a heart attack.

S&M is sitting next to me at the table and keeps a pleasant dinner conversation going punctuated with uproarious jokes and peppered with explicit whispered sexual tips. Slow it down. Don't finish it that way. Mix it up he coaches me.

But Dave never says a word. He just leers and twists his little smirk at me like a guided missile. It does the job. He hasn't said a word to me since he ran away today but something's changed. He's fearless, inviolable and insatiable.

He's grown into his self today. Whatever scared him away earlier seems to have sucked him right back to me. I don't know and I don't care why or what happened. I just know I love him more than air, more than water.

I can't imagine the man sitting across the table from me ever sucking on his fist or whining for his nurse, crying for drugs or getting excited about play money. He's watching me like a prison guard waiting for me to make a move, a guard who knows as soon as I make that move he'll take me down. Cool, dispassionate, controlled.

When the dishes are cleared and the conversation dies, the pauses between words become thick with insinuation. Brandy turns to him and asks gently, "Do you want your shot now?"

He shakes his head and kisses her on the cheek.

"I'm fine," he says. "No more drugs. I ate like a starving dog. I feel fucking good," he laughs and smiles at S&M. "I need a bath."

He breathes in deeply through his nose as if all the bath vapors were already in the air of the room. I can smell them on the sound of his breath.

"Oh, fuck, we're out of here," S&M laughs. "Just don't be crawling into my bed later tonight, son. Take it easy. Pace yourself, man."

Kama Dave walks around the table and pulls my chair back.

"You know what, beautiful?" he whispers. "You really need a bath, you sweet dirty girl. I know just where you can get one with a hundred dollars worth of rose petals and saffron stamens infused in the water with sandalwood oil. I've got a warranty and I guarantee I'll take you straight to heaven."

He takes my hand and leads me up the stairs, locks the bedroom door and starts the bathwater, hot and steaming. He pours in rose, saffron, sandalwood and blue lotus and the steamy scents fill the upstairs with a love fog. The beautiful moonlight pours through the unlocked window onto the unmade bed and spills down on the floor.

He never apologizes or explains, but instead shows me his intentions and desire with his eyes and his smile. He pulls my dress off slowly and puts my hand on his heart and whispers.

"Can you feel me?" he asks. "You have my heart in your hand. I've been such a foolish boy but I'm a man now."

Then he shuts off the bath, strips off his jeans, and we climb into the near scalding water, me lying back on his lap with his arms wrapped around my heart. We just sit and soak and breathe the beautiful erotic scents and I hear him purring like a machine. After a long time he says its time to pull the plug. The water is barely tepid now and I'm half asleep from the rhythm of his heartbeat and breath.

He dries me lightly and leads me to bed, adding more oil to my damp skin, and then he asks softly if he can try again. Please with sugar. Not the belt stuff, he says; he likes it but he doesn't need it tonight because he's—he puts my hand on him and he's fully aroused. I can feel his pulse in my hand. He doesn't need to play now.

He kisses me and bites my lip and sucks my tongue and I remember S&M saying slow it down, mix it up. Don't finish it like that. So I kiss his throat, his heart, his belly and when I put his sex in my mouth this time I go slow and bite a little and listen for his breath and his surprised sighs of pleasure and I keep it going soft and easy like the moonlight. I make it last and last.

When he comes close, I go slower and when he comes to the edge I stop. Then I slide back up his beautiful warm body to his mouth and let him take control. He moans and laughs and takes me straight to heaven. I feel his orgasms coming steadily but he never finishes. Eventually he falls asleep still inside me, locked in my arms, entangled with my soul in the same dream as mine.

All through the night, in and out of dreams, I feel him sending waves of love and pleasure through me. It's dream sex he tells me in the morning. He just invented it for me he says; it never ends. There is no hard and fast ejaculation, just the constant exchange of kundalini prana.

And then I realize S&M had it all wrong about Kama Dave. He's not into straight sex at all; he's into Tantric sex and he's gone far beyond the edge of the physical act into the realm of pure love and intimacy. He's taken my soul prisoner.

†

## NAT

I'm helping Prince make breakfast, baked eggs au gratin over asparagus along with a fresh fruit salad and yoghurt, his usual easy elegant fare. Dave comes in the kitchen looking radiant and hungry and asks if he can help.

"Not much left to do," Prince says offering him some coffee.

"Nat," Dave begs, "I need some work. Can I apprentice with you in the lab? Is there anything I can do to make a little money?"

Dave's never worked a day in his life and I'm pretty sure he hasn't got any marketable skills, but I don't want to discourage him. He's fiendishly passionate about botanical oils, especially the meditatives, aphrodisiacs and sedatives.

I tell him he can work with me but being an apprentice means trading time for knowledge, not money. And since he's under house arrest, he doesn't really need money for anything.

"How about you, Prince," he tries. "What could I do to help?"

Prince laughs at him and says you can't work in the kitchen without a shirt or shoes. Dave frowns and tries another tack.

"How about a loan then?" he asks.

"You have no way to pay me back," Prince frowns. "And anyway I'm saving my money to buy a car."

"Why do you need money, honey?" I ask.

"I want to buy something nice for my wife," he smiles.

"That's sweet," I say. "Maybe you should talk to Sunny. She handles our payroll. She might have an idea for you."

"Prince," he tries again, "I could help you write those love letters. I've got some steaming hot words I can give you."

Prince puts the tray of eggs in the oven and turns around to give Dave his full attention. "Hmm," he says. "I'll bet you know some good words. Write some for me and I'll tell you if I want to buy them. How much money do you need?"

"About $500, I think," Dave says. "It depends. I need to get on the Internet and see how much it costs."

"I couldn't give you more than $50 for some love letters. A $500 love letter would probably spontaneously combust. It would probably scare anyone I sent it to. Maybe you should buy her something smaller. Maybe you should just pick some flowers for her from the forest."

Dave sulks. He hasn't got a penny and he never even noticed it until now. He's always been content with bare feet, jeans and flowers. He picks Prince's book up from the kitchen table and opens to the pictures and frowns. Then he closes it and says, "Fine. I'll write a $50 love letter. Maybe you'll want more if you like it."

Nicky comes into the kitchen and puts her arms around his shoulders and kisses the top of his head. He picks up the book again and shows her a picture.

"Oooh!" she moans, "very rough and sexy and soft all at the same time."

"I knew you'd like that," he smiles. "It's pretty twisted."

She pours herself some coffee and sits at the kitchen table leaning against Dave like a flower stretching towards the sun. I can't imagine her needing any gifts from him other than his sweet smile. Jain smells the baked eggs and joins us at the table.

"No more drugs, Dave?" he wonders. "You just went off the sedatives completely? I'm impressed. What's your secret?"

"I'm sleeping better," he laughs. "I'm not bothered by the planet spinning anymore. I'm starting to enjoy it a little. Actually a lot!"

We dig into the fruit salad and yoghurt and honey while we wait for the eggs to bake. Brandy comes in with a bucketful of jasmine boughs followed by Sim, and Dave gets up to hug them both. Sim looks him in the eye and laughs, "Who the fuck is this guy?" And then he kisses him full on the mouth.

"Good morning, son," he says. "You look good. You look peaceful again. You must have had a good sleep." He grins at Nicky. "Has he behaved?"

"Perfectly," she purrs. "He gets a gold star."

Prince pulls the baking dishes out of the oven and passes them around carefully. "I was wondering about those love letters, S&M," he says quietly. "Am I going to get any?"

"Sure, man," Sim says. "I've got a half dozen for you to start with. Nicky will go over them with you and help you narrow it down to a couple favorites. Nat can give you some good advice as well. There's a ton of them, but I think you'll like the ones I picked."

Prince blushes and smiles and digs into his eggs. "Thanks," he mumbles.

Sim turns back to Dave and snickers, watching him spoon feeding Nicky. "You got it sorted out, Kamadev?" he asks.

"A gentleman doesn't talk about sex in public," Dave scolds.

"*I'm* not a gentleman," Nicky laughs. "You were way off base on the subject, S&M. He's completely into Tantra. He's invented dream sex which goes all night while you're sleeping."

"Aw, shit! Not at the table," Prince moans.

"If you knew how much sex goes on at the table, you'd never cook again," Sim roars. "Food is completely sexy, young man, especially that cherry sauce. You're probably responsible for dozens of orgasms last night."

Prince puts his head down and blushes furiously. I want to hear more about Tantric dream sex, but I don't want to torture the poor boy by talking about it any more at the table. So I just ask Nicky if she'd like to go over the love letters with me in the lab after breakfast.

"Perfect," Sim says. "I've got some personal business with Kama Dave after breakfast. Private yoga lessons, right Dave?"

Dave looks at him confused for a few seconds and then remembers. "Oh, right, the private lessons. I'm all over it, Nim."

†

## S&M

"The first thing you want to remember about a strip tease is it's all about the tease, not the strip."

We're out on the yoga deck behind the pool house with the door locked, completely private. I know the ladies are going to be tied up for hours gossiping about Tantric dream sex and mulling over which of Kama Dave's love letters and marriage proposals are suitable for Prince Albert. We've got all the time in the world.

Dave is going to be a rock star stripper, mainly because he's got that other worldly attitude going for him, like he's just beyond the edge of here and now and can't be touched even if you paid him. But right up front he says something that worries me.

"I need to make a little bit of money, Nim," he whines. "I haven't got a penny."

"Well, hang on. You're not going to strip for money or I'm not even going to teach you. This is supposed to be for love."

"It *is* for love," he moans, "I'm not talking about being a professional stripper. I just want to buy her something nice. I just need a little money to make her happy."

"Oh, you're already making her very, very happy, baby. She doesn't need a present."

"Noooooo," he groans. "I just want to give her this one thing. She didn't even get a wedding present."

"You're the present, honey," I assure him. "She's very satisfied. Trust me. Now pay attention because she's going to go crazy over this and it won't cost you a penny."

"Okay," he nods, "Let's do it. I get it. It's not about the strip; it's about the tease. I like to tease her, Nim."

"Yeah, me too," I say. "That's my specialty. I love to pull on the wings of angels. By the way, that was very powerful stuff you did last night at the table, pulling her hair, not talking to her, playing with the chair, aggressive eye contact. You've got the idea. She loved it didn't she?"

He laughs. "I loved it, too, Nim. It's a good game."

"Cool. The biggest problem you're going to have is you haven't got a lot of clothes to strip off. But you just play with what you've got, like it's not quite on or quite off. You show a little bit and then cover it up; you play with your bits and pieces.

"What you want to do is add some extra toys to your arsenal. You can do a whole lot with just jeans, but you can do much more with accessories. Add the blessing scarf, a belt, your bodybuilding gloves, a hat can rock it really nice, the silk kimono, you see where I'm going? The more the better. I like to use the cop hat. You can borrow it.

"A nice start is to strip off your handcuff bracelet and lock her up so she can't touch you during your act, the tease."

He laughs, "I get it."

"Okay," I say. "Let's start with the porn star walk. You can fuck with her all day long just walking around the house and yard with that. Here's how it's done, like a model walks, one foot in front of the other midline, you can even cross over a little and exaggerate it. The point is to let her know you're walking for her pleasure, to entertain her with eye candy, not just to get across the room. Try it.

"Good job, yeah, it forces you to swing your hips to keep from falling on your face. Okay. Start practicing that around the house. You're going to freak Prince Albert out but it's not really your problem. You're also going to drive Nat crazy, but she's going to have to deal with it. God knows she asked for it.

"Next we're going to work out a routine. And when we're happy with it, you'll invite Nicky to a private show with lights, music, furniture, costume, the whole whack."

We work on his routine for an hour or so with a couple of my kitchen chairs on the deck, a few borrowed pieces of Brandy's clothing, my cop hat and handcuffs and belt and he's good right out of the gate. I'm beaming with pride. I just want to see him make Nicky happy. This is going to be my wedding present to her. Money can't buy it.

But at the end of the lesson, he says he's got to go talk to Sunny about getting on the payroll so he can get some money.

"Hang on, Dave," I say. "I'm telling you this is better than anything you can buy her. I know Nicky. What could you possibly buy for her that's sexier than a strip tease?"

He smiles and his eyes shine. "I showed it to her, Nim. She says it's very rough and sexy and soft at the same time. She wants it very much." And he lowers his voice and whispers to contain his excitement.

"Oh, shit," I laugh. "Why didn't you just come out and tell me, man? Yes, she would like that very much. I could give you an allowance for something like that. Let's go see Sunny and I'll authorize payment from my account. You rock, son."

†

## SUNNY

Sim and Dave come prowling around the office door while I'm working on our accounts, looking like they've just escaped from reform school. Dave's hair is wild and his face is flushed and he walks in with a provocative strut like a porn star, the same way I see Sim parading around the grounds. Sim looks even wilder but they knock politely and behave like perfect gentlemen.

"Sunshine, we'd like to put in an online order. On my personal account," Sim says. "Would you let us use the computer?"

He's the corporate president, so I haven't got a problem with it, although if he were using a business account I'd have to authorize it. I wonder what they're on to now after all the esoteric luxuries, oils and silks the Fire House has been ordering.

Dave doesn't have a clue how to use the computer so Sim gives him a little lesson on how to search for what he needs and when it pops up Dave laughs with joy.

"It's less than $200!" he smiles. "That's perfect."

"Yeah, it's a local store, too. We can get it delivered I'm sure. Let's just phone the order in."

I peek over Sim's shoulder and see the object of Dave's delight: black leather pants.

"Check out the belts, too, Dave," Sim says. "It's cheap enough to get a few more accessories. That braided one with the tie instead of buckle is smart. You won't get hurt that way. And get the bolo necklace with the silver beads on it. It's hot; you can really play with that thing."

He looks up and sees me gaping at the screen and he laughs, "Wedding presents for Nicky. Except they go on him, not her."

"Oh," I say. It's all I've got to say. It's all I want to say.

Sim gets on the phone and puts in the order and then he puts his hand over the receiver and says, "Hell, son. Do you mind if I copy you for a change? I could use all of the above myself."

Dave says be my guest, and Sim gets back on the phone and doubles the order.

"Brandy never had much of a wedding present either. She got kicked out of the honeymoon house while I was going through withdrawals, and she's never complained about a thing."

"Yeah, she's a good girl, Nim," Dave agrees. "You should keep her. Hey, can I look for something else? Love poems?"

Oh. I know just what he wants. I've just been looking at the most beautiful anthology of erotic poetry and I show it to him and print out one I think he might like.

*"Hypnotized by your voice my heart pounds*
*I see your soul and my face burns at the sight*

*Words fail and I can only groan and fall*
*Like a leaf destroyed by your sweet breath*
*Nothing can save me" – Sappho*

"Oh, Sunny," he swoons. "That's a $500 poem. It's much too nice for Prince. It would spontaneously combust and scare anybody away. But I can use it. I know Nicky would love it. Thanks for that!"

"Buy the book," Sim orders. "Buy a copy for yourself, too, Sunny on my account. If you find any more sexy stuff that good, let me know. We can't get enough of it."

He laughs, but I can see he's serious. Both of them are too fast, too wild, too twisted for me to understand, but I can't take my eyes off them as they walk out of the office laughing and swaggering with that sick stripper strut. In fact, I get up from the desk and go to the window just so I can watch them walking all the way across the yard until they're out of sight.

†

NAT

It's nearly sunset when the boys finish drooling over the love letters. Nicky's out on some secret errand and I'm trying to keep my nose out of their business by working in the lab, but the whispers, howls and giggles are driving me crazy. I channel the sexual charge in the air by mixing a beautiful new blend of rose attar, saffron and jasmine with just a hint of vanilla. When I'm happy with it, I bring it into the boardroom and let Dave have a sniff.

"Oh, ouch," he whispers. "That's filthy, Nat. That ought to be illegal. I could use some of that."

"How's this one, Nat?" Prince asks me a little shyly. "She looks very nice."

He shows me a photo of a girl who looks a lot like a younger version of Brandy. She looks about the right age for him but she's got blood red lipstick on her and it bothers me a little, a bit fast for him I think. I put some of the love oil behind his ears and he winces. He's almost as fearful of women as he is homophobic.

"Sweet," I say. "You can't tell by a picture, though. What did she write?"

"Well, it's addressed to Dave, but she's very interested. She's put her phone number and everything in it. Email. Damn, she's got a website even. I think I need to get on the computer and check her out."

"Why not just call her?" I ask. "You can tell a lot more about a person by talking to them."

"No way," he says. "I've got to think about this. Dave will help me write a letter of introduction first. Then we'll see."

"I'm not sure about her, Prince," Dave adds. "I think pink lipstick is a lot sweeter. I like the cinnamon pink pearl. That red stuff looks predatory. Just my two cents worth though."

Prince has got the night off tonight so we've ordered Mexican takeout. When the doorbell rings, I assume it's the food. But when I open the door, I'm nearly knocked off my feet. My first thought is who ordered the hooker?

There's a girl at the door, no more than seventeen, dressed in skin-tight purple leather pants, a little white lace camisole and a red fox fur pillbox hat. She's got hippie beads around her neck, feather earrings, and not a drop of makeup except for the layered mascara. She's definitely not delivering Mexican food.

"Hey," she says. "I've got a delivery for Kama Dave Dixon. House of Leathers. Is he home?"

"Uhhh," is about what comes out of my mouth. "Uhhh, ooofuck. Dave?"

He struts up behind me and smiles at her.

"Oh, come in. Come in," he gushes. "Please."

She looks around and walks into the boardroom with the authority of a CEO. She's got her eyes glued on Dave's hair. She likes him very much I can tell. Prince Albert is nearly choking on air, immobile, frozen in space.

"I'm Dave. This is Nat and our chef, Prince Albert. It's an honor to have you deliver my order personally. Man, I can't wait to get this stuff on. I've never had stuff this nice. How's the leathers feel on? I bet it's fucking sexy."

He puts his hand on her purple leathered ass and she doesn't even flinch. She likes it.

"I had to bring this up myself, Mr. Dixon. I've got your centerfold from the newspaper on my bedroom wall. You fucking rock, Kama Dave. I wrote you a letter."

He blushes. "Oh, I never even read those. I got carried away."

"Oh, sorry. I didn't even introduce myself. My name is Cat."

"Cat. Nice. I'm fucking married but Prince Albert is available. He's a virgin. He's taking my overflow. Do you like cherry sauce? This boy can give you orgasms just by cooking."

She laughs and stares at Prince, sizing him up. He turns cherry red and stares at the top of the table.

"What are you waiting for, Mr. Dave Dixon?" she teases. "Let's rock'n roll."

He grins and takes the box upstairs to try on his new pleasures. Cat sits down at the table across from Prince.

"Chef Virgin Prince," she smiles. "I think you just made my day. What is your house specialty?"

"Uh," he stammers. "Ummm. Ooof. Probably baked eggs. Crème brulé. My crepes are pretty nice, too, with cherry flambé."

"You're into your cherries," she laughs. "What's up with that?"

"They're not too sweet," he says. "They're wickedly tart and they stand up to anything. What a chef really looks for is perfect balance. You need to let all the flavors shine without overwhelming your palate."

"Oh fuck!" Cat swears looking up at Dave strutting down the stairs in his new leather pants, his braided tie belt and bolo necklace. "Oh, kill me now so I can die happy."

Dave smirks at her but he seems a little shy about it, like he's in deep water over his head. "Good enough for Valentine's Day?" he asks.

"Good enough for fucking bigamy," she spits. "Oh Holy Shit. Do you want to get married again, Dave?"

"Probably not," he laughs. "My wife is more beautiful than air and water. You're a sweet girl, Cat, but Nicky is a goddess. And you're much too young for me. I prefer older women."

He gives me such a deep and searing look that I gulp. I can never take back what I did to him and I don't ever want to. His smile is so delicious I can taste him. Then he turns back to Cat and continues.

"But Prince here is pretty interested. You couldn't find a nicer guy his age. He's actually a retired entrepreneur and makes a lot of money as a personal chef. You should grab him before he starts writing love letters to this little girl."

He shows her the photo and she takes it from his hand and tears it in half.

"She's too late, Dave," she laughs.

I'm thinking if the girl with red lipstick was too fast for Prince, the House of Leathers Cat Girl is probably going to wreck his transmission and blow out all four of his tires. The doorbell rings again and this time it's a young Mexican guy with the food so I point him towards the kitchen.

"Um, Cat," Prince sighs, "Can you stay for dinner? I mean I didn't cook it but I'd love to feed you anyway. I'm really happy you came. The chile rellenos are especially delicious."

Cat gets up and goes around the table to sit next to him, leaning into his shoulder.

"Oh, man," she says surprised. "You smell like—God what do you smell like? It's the most beautiful thing." She sucks air and hums with joy at the love oils. "Oh, man. Prince, honey. You smell like happily ever after."

She's got her little fur hat buried in his neck and she's purring up at him when Sim walks in from the kitchen with a burrito in his hand.

"Oh, man, I'm paying you way too much if you can afford a girl like this. Where'd you find the hooker, Prince?"

Prince jumps to his feet and runs into the kitchen to fix a couple plates. He hisses at Sim in passing, "She found me. House of Leathers delivery. Blame Dave."

Dave laughs and says, "I don't know about whores, Nim, but this is how rock stars dress. It's just hot stuff." He shows him Prince's book with the photo of the drummer boy dressed in black leather and lace.

"Oh, sorry, honey," Sim apologizes to Cat. "I was just kidding about the attire. The purple looks good on you." Then he turns to Kama Dave and whistles. "Good thing you're under house arrest, buddy. You could cause a car wreck in that outfit. Where's mine? I'll show you how it's supposed to be done."

Dave points to the stairs and Sim takes his sweet time walking across the room, swinging his hips. Cat nearly falls out of her chair watching him go up the stairs.

"Oh, God. It's really him," she gushes. "S&M. It's really him. OMG! It's horrible," she whispers as soon as he's out of sight. "I mean his back. He's beautiful but the scars are so horrible." And then she blushes and stares at the plate of food Prince put in front of her. "Oh, God, I'm sorry I said that!"

"I don't think it bothers him, Cat," Dave smiles at her. "I don't think he cares how it looks or he'd wear a shirt. I think he kind of likes the way he looks. My wife Nicky says he can have an orgasm just looking in the mirror. It wouldn't hurt his feelings if he heard you. He'd probably just laugh and come again."

And then, speaking of coming, Sim comes down the stairs in his leather pants with the porn step. He's got the braided belt in his hand and he's laughing and smacking his other hand with it. He wraps the belt around his shoulders like a boa, grabs both ends and flexes his biceps with an evil smile.

"Who wants it first?" he mocks looking around at all the open mouths in the room. "Nat," he says looking me coyly in the eyes, "don't I owe you some kind of trouble?"

"No way, boss," I stammer. "Not me. I don't want any trouble today."

"Me! Me!" Cat howls. "I'll take whatever you're dishing out!"

"Nah, honey," he sneers. "You're not a consenting adult. Play with Prince Albert. I've got to go. I think my wife has been a very bad girl today and needs to have some private instruction."

Then he grabs another burrito and struts out laughing like a maniac. He's laughing so hard I can swear I see tears in his eyes.

†

## BRANDY

I see Sim walking across the lawn and right away I know something is wrong. He's dressed in beautiful new leather pants but he's not walking like himself. His head's down and he's dragging a belt in his hand along the grass. He looks up and forces a pathetic smile when he gets close to the front door. He kisses my forehead and hands me a burrito.

"It's still warm," he says. I can see pain in his eyes and his lips are pressed together between his teeth like he's trying to stop his tears.

"Are you looking for a nurse?" I tease him, but he shakes his head no. "I think I need a doctor. I'm fucked."

He goes into the bedroom and straight to the dresser for his sweat pants, the ones he wore when he was so sick, and strips off the leathers without even a tease or a bump and grind. Yeah. I can tell he must really be fucked.

"Can you call Jain for me? It's just bad all of a sudden. I don't know. It only hurts when I breathe. I don't want any narcotics but I need something. It won't stop, Brandy."

"Where's it hurt, honey?" I ask.

"Jain knows exactly where it hurts. The same old shit, except now it's worse."

He lies down on the bed and I pile some pillows under his knees to take the pressure off his lower back. Jain's on the way home from the hospital when I call. He says give him fifteen minutes and he delivers as promised.

"What's up, man?" he says concerned. "What happened?"

"I don't know," Sim whines. "I was feeling so good but now I'm wrecked. My whole back is messed up."

Jain helps him turn over so he can take a look and Sim groans with the pain. Even without touching him, I can see the whole right side of his back is in a spasm all the way down to the lateral insertion at his waist.

"Ouch," Jain says, putting his hands on the hard knotted muscle. "Have you been in the gym today? What did you do to yourself?"

"Nothing," he says. "Nothing much."

"I can give you a steroidal epidural injection if you want. That'll stop it but we'll have to go back down to the hospital for that. There's some special equipment involved. You've already ruled out pain killers and I don't think sedatives are going to do what you want."

"I'm not going back to the hospital," he hisses.

"Well then, we can do the old fashioned treatment, acetaminophen and aminos with massage and rest. But the epidural is good for 3 to 6 months. You should think about it. Did you do anything to aggravate it? I wonder if I need to get the rest of the shrapnel out with surgery."

"Fucking no!" he swears.

"What have you been up to today?" Jain asks him curiously.

Sim just makes a face so I answer for him, "He was giving Dave yoga lessons."

"Okay. Anything strenuous?"

"Actually," Sim winces. "It was strip lessons. For Valentine's Day. But don't mention that to anyone because it's a secret."

"Oh, how sweet, Sim." I tease him. "You're such an incurable romantic. But weren't you giving him fight lessons yesterday, too? There was a little bit of blood."

"The guy got a few lucky punches, Jain," he laughs. "He flattened me."

"You're killing me, buddy. I don't think you need back surgery. Maybe we should consider brain surgery. I'll have Nat come over to help Brandy with some physical therapy. You probably just need a little down time, old man. Don't let him out of bed, Brandy. Ice and massage. You know the drill."

"Nat can't come over right now," Sim says. "She's alone over there with the guys and Prince has got a little Wild Cat clawing at him. I can't stay in bed with all that drama going on next door."

"And you can't keep up with guys ten years younger than you either right now," Jain warns. "I can take over supervising for a few days. Stay in bed and rest. I can handle them."

"Okay then," Sim says. "You can talk to Prince about safe sex so he doesn't get in hot water. Maybe tell Cat it's time to go home. He doesn't have a clue what's up and she came on to all of us pretty hard."

"Me? You talk to him, man."

"You're a doctor. I scare him to death. Dave's giving him sexual advice but he doesn't know the first thing about condoms. He practices control, conservation of bodily fluids. Talk to Prince unless you want a little pregnant rock star moving into your house."

Jain goes back to the Fire House to take over and Nat shows up ten minutes later with fresh flowers, towels and oils.

"You fooled me, boss," she laughs. "I would never have guessed you were in pain after that act. You flattened the room with the floor show. Everyone just calmed down and behaved after you left. Even the Cat was in shock and awe. Now they're just playing games quietly."

"Just sharing the pain, Nat," he says. "I had to laugh to keep from crying like a baby. Sometimes intimidation is the best costume to disguise weakness."

She bends down and kisses his forehead. I usually mind because I know her intentions are pure and simple: to heal him. But everyone wants to help him and they forget he's mine. This time I'm horribly jealous.

"Remember," Nat says, "pain is just weakness leaving the body."

"And that which doesn't kill me makes me a stronger lunatic," he laughs.

"It's nothing serious, Sim," I add. "Nothing a few days in bed won't fix. You might as well enjoy it. Think of it as a little vacation from the asylum. All the rest of the lunatics will still be there when you're better and I can entertain you while you're stuck in bed.

†

JAIN

I'm expecting a teenage orgy when I get back to the Fire House, but instead the kids are sitting quietly around the boardroom table starting a dice game. I pray this is not going to be strip dice.

Prince has the Mexican food in the oven on low and I fix a nice plate for myself before I face imminent sexual mayhem. They're still arguing about the rules and the bets, so I just kick back and absorb without making any judgments. Except I do note that based on the bizarre clothing Cat and Kama Dave are wearing they aren't very likely to be casting their leather pants into a betting pool.

"I know you don't have any real money, Dave," Prince reasons, "but Cat has a lot of it. Why don't you just use the play money and we'll use the real stuff. It's no different from how the government works.

"Real money is just a promissory note based on nothing. It's dirty paper. You just need to sign your initials on the play money so we know it's Kama Dave currency and it didn't just come from the hardware store."

"I'm fine with that, Dave," Cat adds. "You use play money and we'll use real money. Then you get a chance to win some. And if we win some of your play money we can hold it ransom for favors and stuff. Trade or games."

"Alright then," Dave smiles. "I've got $9,000. Prince already has $1,000 of my currency. If he loses badly, I'll buy it back."

"Deal!" They all say in unison. So I'm relieved with that. No clothing involved.

"Want to get in on it, Dr. Jain?" they taunt me. Oh, well why not? I'm a doctor. I'm the CEO of Sunrise. And I'm loaded.

"So here's the rules," Dave says seriously. "These are twisted rules but they're His Rules and they can't be broken. For Shiva dice, we each use two dice. Pairs are the lowest score, but odd number pairs beat even number pairs. So a pair of 1's beats a pair of 6's any day."

"His Rules?" Cat wonders raising an eyebrow.

"They're Shiva's Rules and they can't be broken. The Universe doesn't like everything to be even. Odd pairs are much more interesting.

"But a pair of 1's is actually "2", which is even," Prince complains.

"But not as even as a pair of evens which are evenly separate and together. Those are the rules. But that's also why a pair of anything is the lowest score. The next highest score is a straight, which are two consecutive numbers like 1 and 2, 2 and 3.

"What beats that is a harmonic, a skip: like 2 and 4, or 4 and 6. An odd harmonic beats that. 1, 3 and 5 in any combination beats any of the rest just because those are Shiva numbers.

"Then there's the last provision, double Shiva immunity. With Snake Eyes, you can win but you can't lose any money for two rolls. Pretty simple, huh?"

"Write it down," Prince Albert moans, "so we know you're not cheating."

I remember the night I came home to find the whole house stripped down to nothing because Sim was calling the rules. Then again, as long as everyone is playing by the same rules, all is fair.

Dave writes: Even pairs, odd pairs, straights, even skips, Shiva numbers, and then the highest Shiva double immunity. God help us if Shiva Dice used more than two dice; the rules would probably fill a book.

I haven't got any cash on me so I borrow $1,000 worth of play money from Dave and put my initials on it, telling him I'll settle with real money tomorrow. Dave is blown away now that he has his own bank.

"Fuck yes!" he grins at his new collateral.

By the time Nat comes back from working on Sim, I'm a couple hundred in the hole and Dave is up around $750. Cat has lost $200 and Prince has lost $350. I'm sure it won't hurt Prince because he's got $1,000 in play money equity, but I'm worried about Cat.

"No," she assures me. "It was worth every penny. I make really good commissions on my sales and I can write this off as a business expense. My boss will cover it. I'm sure you'll be great customers.

"But what happened to S&M? Why isn't he playing with us tonight? I would have happily lost $500 to play dice with him. He's a legend."

"He's not feeling well, honey," Nat says. "He's going to be in bed for a couple of days."

"HA!" Dave snorts. "I'll bet he is!"

I start to tell him Sim's back is fucked and he's in a lot of pain but then I remember his reputation as the Sex God of Pleasure Point. Kama Dave worships him and I don't think I want to ruin the S&M legend.

"Maybe even a week," I say instead. "He's very busy. If you need anything, I'm filling in for him. Gym. Fighting. Whatever. And Nat can help you with your yoga."

Kama Dave counts out his cash, very pleased with himself. "Mmm. Fighting might be fun," he says, "but probably just weight lifting with Nicky. Private lessons. That would be very nice, Dr. Jain."

We hear a car pull into the driveway and Dave's eyes turn on like high beams.

"Oh, Nicky!" he purrs. He holds his breath and waits until he hears her key in the lock and the door opens.

She smiles at the little party and says, "Hey, guys, I've got some great yoga books for us from the library. Prince, especially for you, some basic training."

Then Dave gets up from the table and pulls the braided belt out of the loops of his leathers. He puts it around his neck and shoulders, apparently from what Nat tells me later, exactly how he saw Sim do it. He grabs both ends of the belt and flexes his biceps with an evil smile.

"Who wants it first?" he sneers. "Nicky. Don't I owe you some kind of trouble today?"

Nicky drops the books on the floor and faints dead out.

"Ooooh, Dr. Jain," Dave says. "Nicky's not feeling well. Can you help me get her upstairs? She needs to go to bed for a couple of days."

†

## S&M

"Just take it easy and get comfortable, honey," Brandy purrs. "You're going to be my prisoner for a while. You might as well enjoy it. I can read to you if you like or just tease you to death."

I take a deep breath and blow out some of the pain and tension. I haven't spent a lot of time with her since we've been married. We hardly even know each other. Between training the surf team, babysitting Kama Dave, working on the board of directors and trying to rehabilitate my own personal injuries, I've been busy sorting out the Universe and keeping the planets lined up.

Now I think that a time out is going to be a welcome break for me. Maybe it's time I get back to teaching my wife Tantra.

"Teasing me to death?" I laugh. "That sounds interesting. I should have given you strip lessons instead of Dave. Remind me to do that when I'm feeling better."

"I've got something better in mind," she smiles. "Dream sex. Nicky told me how."

"Oh, yeah? In your wildest dreams! I can't move. I don't think dream sex is on the agenda today."

I twist my shoulder a little to see if I've had a miraculous cure but a sharp spasm shoots through me immediately. "Nah," I say. "It's no good."

"Dream sex is perfect for now," she continues. "Trust me. Remember the first Tantra lesson you gave me, how to just wait without it going anywhere? It's just that, a long sexual meditation that doesn't move or finish. It's meant for sleeping and relaxing.

"Nicky said Dave invented it to stop his nightmares but when she told me how it works, I knew it was the exact same thing you taught me when you were sick. It's just a pure Tantric connection. The only thing that moves is your prana.

"She says you can do it all night. I'll bet we could go a couple days." She winks at me and gives me a very twisted little smile. She's got something there. If that's all she's talking about—man, I think—it sounds beautiful.

"But just to make you feel safe and secure—" she gets up and takes the police handcuffs off the shelf and swings them in front of me with a questioning look.

"Oh, all right," I smile. She knows what I like. I'm starting to think this is the best thing that's happened to me in a long time. Screw my back. Maybe I'll get a real honeymoon now.

She cuffs my wrists to the bed headboard, but just as I'm getting a nice sexy buzz going, Brandy starts getting pretty dark, pretty kinky and I start getting nervous about the whole thing.

"I like it when you're hurt, Sim," she purrs, "so I can take care of you and fix you. I want to help you, baby.

"You're a very sick boy. You've been very wild and rough and I need to just quiet you down so I can care for you."

The hair on my neck stands up and my heart jumps when she pulls a hypodermic needle out of the bedside table and smiles.

"You've been much too busy and I knew you were going to hurt yourself again. Let me just soften you up and quiet you down. You need a nurse to take care of you for a few days."

"Hang on, baby!" I warn her. "What the fuck is that? I'm not sick. Jain said I don't need any shots, just some rest and ice."

"Right," she purrs, "I'm going to help you rest. This will make you very soft and comfortable. Kama Dave loved it."

"The anti-psychotics? No thank you. Don't get near me with that stuff."

She's pretty strong for a little nurse though and, with the help of the cuffs, she pins my shoulder down and gets the needle into a vein. And I can't fight her because of my back. She's scaring me. She's drugging me!

"Poor sick boy," she says. "I need to fix you. I got straight A's in nursing school. I know how to make you feel really nice."

Oh, man, my mind starts slipping out from my head and I see her spin. She's given me a huge dose. I like control. I like consciousness and I'm losing everything.

I thought I taught her how to behave herself! She's taking control of the Universe. She's trampling me like Kali dancing on Shiva's body.

As I'm losing consciousness I think about the story of Bluebeard and wonder with a horrible chill if I married a serial killer. Who is she really? She said she likes me to be hurt.

She fell in love with me when I was bleeding to death on the beach. She raped me and married me when I was in intensive care and I'd only met her a few days before. Fucking black widow, I think, femme fatale, as she climbs in bed with me and holds me tight, whispering.

"You're mine, baby. I'm going to take care of you now. You're a very sick boy."

She starts kissing me long and deep and I feel all four of her hands everywhere all over me, taking me where she wants to go. She promised me dream sex, but I'm getting a horror substitute instead – nightmare sex.

I'm not nearly as sick as she is, I think as I go under.

†

## BRANDY

It's easier to ask for forgiveness than to get permission. I know he would never allow this if I asked but on the other hand, he probably won't remember any of it.

He's been teaching me control, but he hasn't taken enough time to help me with my lessons. I'm tired of trying to control myself; I'm more interested in controlling him.

I know he knows things, and he likes things that I don't understand. But I'm a creative girl and I can teach him things he's never dreamed in his wildest imagination.

I have a lot of lorazepam left over since Dave quit taking it and no one seemed to notice. No one asked me to return it to the Ice House pharmacy. No one seems to know that the anti-psychotic sedative is a benzodiazepine, one of the most popular class of date rape drugs.

But I know. I didn't miss a beat in nursing school. And I can't help myself. I love him, but he's so controlling, so tough and wild I can't get close enough to him. 'His way or the highway,' Nicky warned me. 'A very kinky boy,' she said. As the drug takes effect, it knocks the kink right of him.

I see fear in his eyes but then he disappears into oblivion and all that's left is his compliance and animal appetite. When I kiss him, his mouth responds willingly. When I touch him, his cock throbs eagerly. I know, I know it's rape, but he's my husband and he's been holding out on me.

I know exactly how much to give him to incapacitate him without debilitating him or killing him. I know exactly how long I have before he comes back. The first time I raped him it took 10 minutes and he laughed at me. I've got about 10 hours this time, and now I know exactly what I'm doing and how to drive him.

And I know he probably won't remember much of anything when it's over. Too bad, because I bet he could get to like this very much, so much better than playing kinky S&M games with Nicky and Nat. I'm reinventing kink.

He taught me enough Tantra that I know how to extend sex indefinitely, long and slow, and I've got complete control now. I take him inside me, pulling his head back by his hair and cover his mouth with mine. He smiles and purrs, doped and willing, and lets me drive for a change.

†

## S&M

The phone rings a hundred and eight times before I can get my hand out there. It's Nat. I'm so happy to hear her voice I say, "NaNaNad! Heeeuu?" and then I fucking fall out of bed onto the floor.

It's pretty cozy on the floor, rock solid and spacious and I find a vertical plane and a corner and tuck myself into a little box-like shape and I fit perfectly in a wedge between the bed way up there and the wall in a perfectly safe package at the corner of floor and table. Funny, I smell like soap. I go back to sleep.

†

## NAT

I'm ready to quit. You know, it's a nice idea, alternative health, but the only way it works is if the patient embraces healing. Who am I fooling? I thought Sim could teach me and I thought he could help me heal myself.

I dreamed of working with the legendary mad Tantric teacher, collaborating on his mission to destroy all of humanity's pain and suffering, the bodhisattva vow to bring enlightenment to the whole planet or to die trying. But maybe he's gone too far into the deep end.

Kamadev has already torn my heart apart. Jain is a beautiful lover, but he hasn't come close to tying the knot even though he proposed. And Sim—well, Sim is burning both ends of his candle.

He was supposed to be my mentor but right now he seems completely maniacal and confused.

When he came downstairs in his leathers smacking his hand with his belt and asked me if I wanted trouble, I was shocked. I don't want trouble from him! I want guidance, leadership and inspiration. I want to work with him, not get worked over by him.

I'm ready to resign. I call his house and no one answers but I let the phone keep ringing like a mantra. Over and over and over and then suddenly I hear a giggle and "wha?"

"Sim? It's Nat. Can we talk?"

And I hear nonsense slurring over the phone.

"NaNaNad, HeeeeU?" And then I hear a crash.

I just want to lie down on the floor and die but he's my boss and deep in my heart I love him. I ask Jain to come with me and we walk over to the pool house. No one answers the door, but it's open.

The bed is a mess with the sheets spilling onto the floor but it's empty. No one answers our calls. Jain goes out to check the deck but there's no one there. And then I notice feet. He's tucked in like a small package between the bedside table, the wall and the bed, naked, unconscious and defenseless.

I bend down to shake him and the first thing I notice that's wrong is he smells like soap. He's been freshly bathed. Normally he smells like Palo Santo and Sandalwood.

He opens his eyes and laughs. "Awful out. Awful."

"What, honey?" I ask. He's stoned out of his mind.

Jain comes back in the room and says, "Aw, shit!"

"Aw yah," Sim slurs. "Aw ful. Outta bed."

Jain picks him up and puts him back in bed and covers him. "Shit, Sim. You fell out of bed?"

"Ya. Aw ful out," he laughs.

Jain looks at his pupils and then checks his arm and sees the needle mark and swears.

"I can only imagine," he says. "Sim doesn't know how to shoot up. What the fuck happened here? Where is his wife?"

"Where's Brandy, Sim?" I ask.

"War she?" he slurs. His speech is pathetic. It breaks my heart to see such a powerful man incapacitated and helpless. "War?" he repeats.

Jain is already on the phone to the office and Mack says the nurses are gone on errands. Brandy and Sunny left over an hour ago.

I guess it's not a good day to resign. I tell Jain I'm happy to just sit with him and make sure he doesn't fall out of bed again. I'll wait until he recovers.

It scares me how closely he resembles Kama Dave in this state, detached, naïve and childish. The beautiful domineering master of the Universe is reduced to rubble. I almost wish he would regain his composure again, jump back into his leathers and snarl at me with his belt.

I'll appreciate it more the next time I see it.

"My guess," Jain suggests, "is an overdose of lorazepam. Brandy doesn't make mistakes like that so maybe she had to put him down for some reason. Maybe he got out of line. I can't see that happening though. It doesn't make sense.

"It's a heavy drug and he wouldn't even know what hit him. But those are the symptoms, slurred speech, loss of balance and cognition. I can't believe she left him like this."

"She cleaned him up very nicely before she left, Jain," I say. "That really bothers me. Guilt?"

"I don't want to think about it, Nat," he says. "I don't want to go there. That's between Sim and

Brandy. Stay with him and call me if you need me. I'll be in the office with Mack."

†

S&M

I wake up and Nat is sitting in the chair with her eyes closed. There's something dark and ominous in the room, something terrifying and sexy at the same time but I don't know what it is. I'm afraid and turned on at the same time. I wonder what day it is.

"Nat," I whisper. "What happened?"

My stomach aches and my head throbs and I feel like I've been—uh, fucked to death. My usual high voltage libido has been siphoned off and there's nothing left of me. My sexual radiance is snuffed.

"Nat, what did you do to me?" I gasp.

"Me? Holy shit, boss. I haven't touched you. We found you on the floor and I'm just making sure you don't fall out of bed again."

"What?" I grimace. "Where are my damn handcuffs when I need them? I thought I was safe here."

I look around the room and the shelf is empty. I remember—nothing. Kama Dave and Prince had a little girl friend and I simply dropped dead after that.

But there's something very troubling in my loins, as if—no, not Nat. It couldn't be. Shit, Nicky? That would be the day. And certainly not the little well behaved nurse I married. I feel as if I've been fucked by the whole universe in my sleep, revisiting hundreds of karmic ghosts from my promiscuous teenage excesses. I wonder if I'm even now.

"Would Abhyanga help ground you a little, boss? Is there anything I can do to help?"

"Nah, I don't think I want anybody touching me right now. I feel kind of strange."

"Do you remember what happened? Did you take any drugs, Sim?"

"I remember my back hurt and I went to bed. That's it. Where're my fucking clothes? I need to get out of here."

"I think your jeans are still in Dave's room. You left our house yesterday wearing leathers. You want those?"

The thought of putting leather pants on horrifies me. Something very bad happened. I don't want to touch them. She picks my sweats up from the floor and offers them to me. "Or these might be more comfortable," she says.

I take them and pull them on under the covers.

"Yesterday? Where have I been?"

"Jain told you to stay in bed for a few days. I thought you were resting, but when we came by earlier you were a zombie, extremely stoned. Maybe I can help you piece it together. Do you want to talk about it?"

I don't. I need to get out of here. I just bolt past her in spite of her entreaties, out the front door and around the side of the pool house to the forest trail. I can hear her calling after me, but I can't be stopped. I keep on the trail until the house is out of my view and then I cut through the brush straight down the mountainside.

Nearly an hour later I find myself on the edge of a ravine that drops into a beautiful stream. I climb carefully down the side and lower my body into the icy water, lying back so I'm fully immersed in it.

It's late in the afternoon and the air is crisp, but the stream caresses me as I listen to its murmuring mantras. I hear it singing quietly and carefully, and my panic subsides. I tip my head back so my ears are underwater and I listen to strange watery voices whispering down from the top of the mountain as the stream flows to the ocean.

I am the ribbon that ties the mountain to the sea. My mouth spreads with joy and I watch the beautiful window of the sky through the treetops: empty sky waiting for me to pour my soul into its embrace.

After a long time, the sky window turns black. I watch the Milky Way emerge and colored meteors streak around its edges: blue, red and yellow flames across the night sky. I stay in the arms of the water until the moon fills the window and the stars disappear and then I climb up the banks of the stream and heat my body with Agni-Prasana, the Breath of Fire.

Besides creating heat, this kundalini breath recharges my nervous system and purifies my blood. Contracting and expanding pressure on my nerves and glands causes them to fire and my seminal fluids, what's left of them, will release back into the bloodstream and restore my radiance. It might take days or weeks, but I know how to do this, how to get my Shiva back.

Maybe I should have never given up celibacy. I thought there was enough of me to go around after all this time, but now I'm drained and miserable again like I was when I was eighteen.

†

## BRANDY

My first time with Sim, he explained to me that he wasn't much impressed or interested in straight sex, that he enjoyed something a little more interesting and esoteric. I remember him saying old school sex doesn't last very long and usually takes more out of you than it gives you.

But I've been getting impatient with him. Tantric sex is so different and requires such a high level of control and awareness that I find it frustrating, even though it's extremely erotic and pleasurable. I want to *get* somewhere, to finish it off.

Now, I'm horrified at what I've done. I finished it off all right. I played with him for hours and used all the methods he taught me to extend it, to circumvent ejaculation, but in the end I was so out of control, I made him come hard over and over.

After the third time, when I was completely exhausted and sated, I felt a wave of remorse come over me harder and bigger than any orgasm a woman could ever hope to have. And I felt like Eve who tasted the apple and got kicked out of Paradise. I had to get out of there fast.

I cleaned him up nicely with a hospital bed bath and left him to sleep it off. There was no one I could confide in but Sunny. I know she never approved of Sim and thought I was crazy to marry him, so I hoped I could count on her sympathy.

Driving down the mountain towards the coast, she's laughing, telling me about the boys using her computer to order all their sexy leather accessories and she swears, "Damn, Brandy, those boys are much too wild for anyone's safety. They ought to be handcuffed and taught some manners."

And then I just start crying, sobbing out of control. She pulls the car over at the next turn out and puts a hand on my shoulder.

"What?" she asks. "What did that SOB do to you now?"

"Oh, Sunny," I moan. "What have I done? I handcuffed him and doped him and I don't think I taught him any manners at all. I just abused him. I'm so sorry. I lost control. I don't know what I should do now."

"Oh my God, Brandy. What were you thinking?"

"I was thinking how delicious he is and how utterly impossibly domineering. I just wanted to take care of him again, to make him depend on me. He's driving me crazy, Sunny."

"Yeah, I warned you, girl friend. I told you he was dangerous for you. Pretty poison. But that won't help you now. You're in it up to your eyes. What did he say?"

"He was unconscious. When I left, he was still out. I don't know if he'll remember. Lorazepam is a date rape drug. I might be okay. I don't know. Could you find out for me if I'm in trouble? Can I go home again?"

"You need a time out, Brandy. Let's go down to the wharf and have lunch and a few drinks and chill out. Then we'll call Mack and innocently inquire. It might just blow over."

I nod and dry my eyes and we continue driving down the mountain. Around some of the turns we catch an eyeful of ocean dancing like diamonds under soft rivers of fog.

I remember the first time I laid eyes on Sim strutting bare-chested down the beach like a god. He didn't speak to me until he was hurt. He would have ignored me completely. I'm sick. I didn't know I was this twisted.

A drink might take the edge off. Fresh Crab Louis salad and a bottle of Sauvignon Blanc might fix me. Maybe it will all blow over.

It's a beautiful afternoon and the surf is up. From the restaurant on the wharf we can see surfers dropping into the big groomed swell breaking like machinery around the headlands. Far above the green glass hundreds of spectators line the cliff watching the spectacle.

Sim would kill to be here. My stomach sinks at the thought of him and the sight of the crab salad but once I taste the wine, my appetite roars back. My god the sex with that man! Why can't I just put my guilt away and savor what I had: hours without restraint, unless you count his handcuffs?

I pour another glass of wine and remember how he walked across the lawn dragging his belt, dressed in leathers, hurt and coming back to me for help. Oh, Sim, I think, you've undone me.

"Sunny?" I whine. "I'm afraid I'd do it again if I get the chance. I just can't get enough of him."

"Right. Sexual perversion is contagious. You're definitely terminal, Brandy. I saw this coming from the day you took your shoes off."

She laughs a little grim reaper laugh and I know she's right. I'm sick and there isn't a doctor or nurse alive who can cure me.

I rip into the sough dough bread and slather it with unsalted butter to balance the sweet briny crab. I'm ravenous. I think about Prince and wish he could taste this and cook for us like this, and then I just think about—Prince. Eighteen years old. Oh, shit. I rip into some more bread and drown it in Sauvignon Blanc to erase my errant thoughts.

"Brandy," she warns, "I think you might be losing the plot, honey. Why don't you talk to Nat when we get home and see about some therapy?"

"Fine. Fine. Fine," I say. I need help but right now I just need to know how much damage I've done. "Call the office."

Sunny calls the pool house but there's no answer after a dozen rings, so she calls the office.

"Hi, Mack," she purrs. "I'm just down on the beach having lunch with Brandy and I missed you. How are things?"

She listens and her face drains. Her eyes are on me. My fork is halfway between plate and mouth, and my appetite is lost.

"We're on the way," she says and hangs up.

"Brandy. He's um—gone."

†

DJ

Before the sun rises, I'm waiting. A soft gray light creeps into my bedroom and I can hear the song birds serenade the new morning. I've been sleeping inside her but I don't want to wake her until she's ready. I wait for something more beautiful than the rising sun, more intimate than her naked body twisted and nearly braided around mine. I wait.

Then I hear a sharp intake of her breath and a sigh and it happens. First one eye opens and then the other and I'm diving into a deep pool of bottomless emerald eyes, peering into her soul. Aw, Nicky. I come so hard at that my heart skips.

She feels it and laughs and purrs and pulls my hair and then rolls over on top of me and shows me some old school moves, slowly with reverence and respect. She takes me all the way to the edge a dozen times and makes me come but she never finishes me. The way we make love, it never ends.

By the time the sunlight pours through the window, I'm ravenous. There's a beautiful scent of pancakes and coffee drifting up the stairs. I pull on my leather pants and tie the fringe belt neatly through the loops. She puts on her long green dress and saffron silk kimono and then she stares at me and puts her fingers back in my hair.

"Something else, baby Dave," she smiles. "Some little sweet decoration."

She takes a tiny jar of Tiger Balm out of the bedside table and dabs a dot of it between my eyebrows. I feel its heat and smell its pungent aroma and take a look in the mirror. As powerful as it feels, it's barely visible, just a faint golden smear on my forehead.

"Divine perfection," she purrs and she takes my hand and kisses the Om tattoo above my knuckles and then the tips of my fingers. If it weren't for the seduction of pancakes I would never be able to get out of bed.

Nat is sitting at the boardroom table and Jain is pacing the room on the telephone, listening and not saying much. He hangs it up and turns to her anxious eyes and shakes his head.

"Good morning," she says cheerfully when she sees us. Her smile is forced and her voice is staged. I smell a whiff of trouble underlying the steaming pancakes that Prince piles on the table with wild blackberries and maple syrup.

"What's wrong, Nat?" Nicky asks. "You look worried, honey."

Nat shakes her head and starts playing with her food and then throws a sharp warning look at Jain.

"Look," he says. "It won't hurt to tell them. Maybe they can help." He sits down across from us and looks dismally at his empty plate.

"Sim took off," he says. "He was—um, upset about something and he went down the backside of the mountain yesterday. When he didn't come back last night, Sean issued an APB for him. So far, nothing.

"I'm thinking of going down and looking for him myself this morning, Dave. Maybe you'd like to come."

I remember my list. Sim said don't go down into the forest with Jain or Nat, just with him or Nicky. But that was months ago when Jain was angry and jealous. Since then he's been very sorry. I've counted 67 apologies so far and pretty soon I'm going to forgive him for beating me up.

But right now, my feet are starting to sweat, my skin crawls and my jaw is tight. My teacher, my father, my guardian. Where is he?

"Ouch, Dave!" Nicky groans as I crush her hand. I didn't mean to. She puts her arm around me and squeezes my shoulder. "We'll find him, baby. I know he's fine. I know my boy better than anyone. He's probably meditating under a rhododendron tree.

"What happened, Jain?"

"I don't have all the facts," he mumbles. "Nat was with him."

"I'm guessing it was a lovers' quarrel," Nat sighs. "Brandy didn't tell me much but she's coming to see me after breakfast. You've known Sim much longer than I have, Nicky. Do you want to help me with this?"

She says yes so that will leave Jain and me alone in the forest. I sit back in my chair and size him up. He watches me watching him and shakes his head.

"I'm sorry, man," he says. "If you don't want to go, I understand."

"Sixty-eight," I say. "We're getting there. I'll go with you. I know how to fight now," I sneer at him. He hangs his head and apologies for the 69th time.

†

## NAT

When Jain and Dave leave, Nicky and I help clear the table and give Prince a hand cleaning up in the kitchen. I don't want to talk in front of him, so I wonder out loud if he has anything he wants to do today.

"Have I!" he snorts. "Cat asked me to go to the Blues Festival this afternoon. But it's not just blues, there're a lot of rock bands, too. I can be back in time to cook dinner if you don't mind something simple."

"Don't worry about it, honey," I say. "Our boss isn't around right now and we'll be fine with sandwiches."

He smiles but then blushes. "Is he still in bed? It's been three days now!"

"No, he's out. He's just taking a little time off. Enjoy yourself, but behave, okay?"

"Sure. Thanks," he winks. "I'll keep her out of trouble, Nat. Dr. Jain told me how."

He goes back to his room to get ready and comes out twenty minutes later looking like a little dope dealer. He's got a flashy black and silver jersey on with a black doo rag on his head. At least he's not wearing his jeans around his ass like some of the kids do these days. There's no underwear showing and no jewelry. He smiles a little shyly at us as we compliment him but as soon as there's a knock on the door, he bolts for it and disappears.

I make some fresh black tea and sit back down with Nicky at the table and breathe deliberately, long and slow.

"What's going on with S&M, Nat?" she wonders with dark concern. "It's not like him to take off. If he were quarreling with his wife, he'd have no problem correcting her. He's an alpha male, no bones about it."

"You'd think so. But maybe he didn't have a choice."

Brandy comes in the back door and looks at us cautiously. "Nat? Is it a good time?"

"Sit down, Brandy. Nicky's going to talk with us too if you don't mind. I know you trust her and she knows your husband better than any of us."

"Oh, God, Nicky," she moans and starts sobbing pitifully. She sits at the table and buries her head in her arms. This time I'm glad we don't have the whole house here to do group therapy. I'm glad all the boys are gone.

Nicky isn't shy in the slightest and she digs her teeth into the subject without flinching. "Stop it, Brandy. Start at the start. How in hell did you ever marry him?"

Brandy picks her head up and gasps at the heartless tone and the crying stops short. "He never told you?" she sniffs.

Nicky squints one eye and glares at her. "He was celibate the last time I saw him – before I came here. He was my boyfriend but he is as kinky as they come. He was never going to get married."

"But he teased me, Nicky!" she groans. "He was an awful terrible tease. He still is. He's worse than ever. Oh, God, the leathers and the handcuffs and the – "

"Damn," Nicky swears. I have the feeling she has some much more powerful words in mind but she's holding back on us.

"All that Tantric sex," Brandy groans, "all that intimate foreplay that lasts forever and goes nowhere – he's just driving me crazy, Nicky," she pleads for mercy and understanding.

I'm just staying out it. Intake is the most powerful tool a therapist has.

"You don't get it, Brandy," Nicky snarls.

"You said it!" Brandy sobs bitterly. "I don't get it. He loves to play but he's holding out on me! I'm his wife."

"No. I don't mean you don't get sex, I mean you don't get where he's coming from. Hasn't he taught you anything? Hasn't he explained to you what he likes?"

"Um – yes, he's been teaching me, but Nick, he's leaving out the best part. I mean he's not taking care of business, do you understand?"

Nicky drops her head and studies her fingernails and pushes out a few deep sighs. And then she mutters under her breath so that I barely hear her voice:

"*Do not give what is holy to the dogs; nor cast your pearls before swine, lest they trample them under their feet, and turn and tear you in pieces.*"

Then raising her voice to an intimidating whisper she growls, "The best part? The *best* part?"

Silence drops like a bomb in the room. Brandy's eyes are wild and wide and her mouth is open. I can see her mind racing in circles inside her head as she digests her thoughts.

"Which part would that be, Brandy?" Nicky continues with a little hiss. "The orgasm or the ejaculation?"

Brandy is speechless and she turns to me for defense. I understand her confusion.

"Maybe you should have married a straight man, Brandy," Nick continues. "God knows I told you so. You don't even know him."

I try to break the tension in the room. "You could have found a man like Jain," I laugh. "He's so straight it hurts. I'm trying to teach him a little Tantra, but I don't really mind straight. It's probably better for a woman's health."

"Physical health, Nat. Not necessarily spiritual," Nicky corrects me. "Sure there are a lot of beautiful chemicals in a man's seminal fluids but they're just as good for him to store up as they are for our pleasure. We produce a lot of our own. You don't have to drain the poor man to make love with him."

I know she's right, and that's exactly why Brandy is so hungry for him. Seminal fluid contains anti-depressants as well as chemicals that increase affection and induce sleep: estrone, oxytocin, cortisol, thyrotropin, melatonin and the well-known mood-booster seratonin. The sperm is just along for the ride.

I explain to her how a Tantic yogi conserves his seminal fluids to increase his pure sattvic energy. I tell her the journey is much more important than the destination and that Tantra is more about traveling than arriving.

"And Jain?" she asks.

"He's a hyrid," I laugh. "He has the best of both worlds. He likes the ride but he knows when and where to get off." I like the metaphor. Maybe we should trade, I think and then immediately think the better of it. I wouldn't know where to begin with a man like Sim. He would tear me to pieces.

"And Dave?" she looks at Nicky curiously.

"Kamadev? The God of Love? Hardly," she laughs. "He's not interested in ever finishing. He doesn't like to give it up. He just keeps coming.

"But that doesn't bother me in the least. He can rock'n roll for hours. I don't think you appreciate what you've got Brandy."

†

## JAIN

I'm not sure if it's rougher for me or Dave going down the forest trail behind the pool house where I beat him senseless, but after a minute or so I realize it's me.

"Man, I fucked it up, Dave," I plead, trying to shake off the brutal memory. "I wasn't even engaged to her then. It was her choice. I'm so sorry, man."

And he laughs. "Seventy times! Enough is enough. I forgive you, Jain. Nat loves you. We never had anything going more than educational—stuff. Sim asked her to teach me. And she was—compassionate. Not like Nicky. Not like love."

My blood boils anyway at the thought of them together. I'd like to knock his teeth out of his jaw but I think it through. He's just another man like me, smaller, younger, and—I hate to say—prettier but there you go. I can't blame her.

I don't know the terrain at all, so we stick to the path. I cringe as we pass through the grove and I remember the brutality, the hatred and the blood. I breathe deep, like Nat taught me. I inhale love and exhale hate. And then I reverse it with that deeply powerful Tibetan healing practice she taught me. I inhale darkness and exhale light.

I apologize again.

"Seventy-one," he laughs. "I'm not taking any more from you! You're finished, doctor. You have to start all over again with something else if you want to keep groveling."

I stop on the path, not to start new trouble between us but to simply marvel at the young being walking beside me. He's present but he's removed.

"Thanks," I say. "Thanks for the forgiveness, buddy."

Just as he has forgiven me, I let it go, too. As I do, I feel a flood of joy fill me. Why have I been waiting? I resolve to marry her before the day is over.

Something in Dave's voice, his demeanor, his smile, reminds me—and then I realize *everything* in his demeanor reminds me—of Sim. He was psychotic but now he's a simple mirror of his teacher. He could easily be institutionalized, but there's something purer, more enduring and endearing in both of them than sanity.

And then I wonder, is Sim a mirror of psycho Dave right now. Where are you, buddy?

We drop deeper into the forest and see things beautiful and sparkling, waterfalls and dripping flowers. The trail goes nearly vertical. There's no sign of Sim and no answer to our calls.

We walk for hours, down to the end of the trail where it cuts off at the highway. We can see the ocean in the distance, dancing like a diamond in the afternoon sunshine, the fog rolling back in like a blanket tucking the coast in bed for the evening. I know he's down there and I have a feeling he's safe.

"Come on, buddy," I tell Dave. "Let's go home."

We scramble up the embankment to the highway, cross over and start walking back up the long road home. Dave sticks his thumb out with each passing car, but they whiz by ignoring us.

And then I hear a siren flash on and off for a second and turn to see the lights of a cop car pulling up on the shoulder behind us. Sean gives a big grin and waves for us to climb in.

†

## BRANDY

I'm stunned by her venom. My God, she hates me because I don't love him the same way that she loves him. I can feel it like a knife in my belly. I don't know him like she does.

What is the difference between love and lust I wonder? I saw him parading his beautiful body down the beach, twisting his smile and all but dancing with his exotic strut. Sexy, sexier, sexiest. That's all I saw. I saw him on me, under me, in me, with me, by me.

My heart has been ripped out of my chest now and I realize my Sim, my husband, isn't this boy toy, this physical instrument built to please me. No matter how beautiful and alluring the packaging, it's just Maya, the illusion of a man, that I loved.

I remember Dave's words now: 'I was in love with the frosting but I didn't know there was cake inside.'

'How would I know?' he used to cry pitifully whenever his world lost focus. 'How would I know?'

I feel sick as I push myself away from the table and hiss at her. "Fuck you, Nicky!" I hurl the words at her. I've never said that kind of thing before but the pain is brutal and I've got no defense now.

I run into the kitchen crying and tear through the drawers looking for something lethal. Butter knifes, forks, spoons, what fucking kind of kitchen is this? I scream in rage and frustration. And then I remember the little professional ex-dope dealer chef rolling up his knife kit at the end of every meal.

It's a stupid professional kitchen. I can't hurt myself here. Nat follows me in and grabs both my hands and holds me still. I try to break away from her but she's too powerful. When I look into her eyes, I feel a sudden helplessness wash over me like laundry releasing dirt in pure water.

I can't even cry now; my pain is overwhelming and I collapse in her arms shaking uncontrollably. I feel her hands behind my back on my heart as she holds me tight and waits patiently for me to breathe. When I finally take a long deep breath, she lets go of me and opens the kitchen door without a word.

We walk out into the sweet morning air and sunshine and she follows me home, across the lawn, past the gym and the sofa and the pool, past the Ice House with it's surgery and drugs, through the honeymoon bedroom and out onto the yoga deck overlooking the forest and the whole damn creation—overlooking Sim, somewhere out there in the Universe.

She never says a word but sits with me on the bare wood of the deck and we listen to the late morning wind as it shifts onshore.

†

## S&M

I don't sleep all through the night. The stars are too brilliantly entertaining and I swear I've seen at least a dozen extra-terrestrial ships winking at me. I haven't got a watch. It's a joke to me if you need a machine to tell you what time it is.

Time is my prisoner and I love to torture her in the dungeon of my soul. I can always open the door and inquire and find out exactly what time it is.

"Now," she'll scream. "I already told you. It's fucking now."

Mid-way through Vata time, about 4am by sun time I reckon, I pull my feet under me for a formal meditation and chant internal mantras. *Om Triyambakam Yajamahe.* Behold the soul and lingam of the three-eyed Shiva within myself.

Before I sink into the deepest meditation I flick the flies of consciousness aside. I think of Kama Dave, my love, my son, my student. As the story goes, Shiva opened his third eye and burned Kamadev alive because Dev shot him full of love arrows and tempted him to look at Parvati sexually. Later Shiva realizes his error and resurrects Kamadev, but I learn by his mistakes – so I won't bother killing anyone over sex.

But I smile. *Om Triyambakam Yajamahe.* Shiva is the erotic deity of both sex and celibacy. He goes both ways, the Divine porn star. He fathers 48,000 children one weekend, but practices celibacy for a thousand years. Shiva shrines throughout the world are built around the lingam, the phallic sculpture which devotees like to rub with milk and honey. May I bring his energy into the world. Om Namah Shivaya.

I dive down into meditation. Turn off the body. Om. Listen. Turn off the pranic energy. Om. Listen. Turn off the mind. Om. Listen. Turn off the experience. I hum with it. I turn the world with it. What time is it anywhere? Where is it anyway? Who am I? Om Namah Shivaya. I am Shiva the Nataraj, the cosmic dancer. The stream below me tinkles and harmonizes Om. I'm lost right where I want to be.

When I return the sun is winking at me through the treetops. My legs are numb and I massage them gently and then get to my feet. There's no terrain here flat enough to do an asana practice of Surya Namaskar, sun salutations, but there's always foothold enough to do a simple tree pose.

I stretch my hands up to the invisible stars, the blank blue canvas of sky, and fill my lungs with forest air. I focus my gaze, my drishti, on my fingertips and exhale, but something else caches my eyes and they drift to a needle mark on my arm.

Suddenly I remember everything. I feel her next to me, hungry, ravenous, starving Kali biting the heads off men, trampling my poor body under her feet. I hear her whisper in my ear, "You poor sick boy. I like it when you're hurt so I can take care of you. You've been too wild and I can soften you up."

I remember her taking the hypodermic needle out of the bedside table and sticking it in my arm and I see her smile with anticipation and lust. Fuck. I'm going to kill that woman!

†

DJ

"I was just coming up to see you, buddy," Sean grins. "We still haven't found Sim. Crys is down at the beach house in case he shows up there. I wouldn't be surprise if that's were he's headed."

Jain's sitting in the cage in back, but Sean let's me sit up front with him so I won't freak out with all the bad memories. No one speaks for a while and then Sean glances over at me and smiles.

"Wow, Dave. Pretty flashy stuff there. Where'd you get those leathers?"

"Dad. Um—Sim bought them for me. For Nicky. She really likes them."

His smile widens. "Nicky, man. Anything for Nicky. She's a solid gold bomb, Dave. You must have done something right. How's she doing?"

"Perfect," I say. "No complaints. I'm going to keep her."

"Nice job, Dave," he says. "She's good for you. You're not as nervous as you used to be. And you and Jain are getting along okay?"

Jain laughs, "I've been officially forgiven today, Sean. I hope it's okay that I took him off the grounds to look for Sim. Under supervision of course."

"I'm not mentioning it, Jain. Technically, he needs police supervision to leave Sunrise, but I'm here now."

The radio crackles and we hear a report, suspect apprehended on Highway One for vagrancy. Claims to be the APB target but doesn't fit the description.

Sean picks it up and asks, "This is Officer Banks. Steven Mack? Have you got him?"

"We got somebody, Sean, but he's a mess. He's half naked and covered with mud. I thought Mack was a rich guy, clean cut. This one has no money, no ID and he looks like a tramp. He says he's a corporate president. He's mad. I'm taking him in for vagrancy."

"No, hang on a minute. Can I talk to him?"

The radio is silent for a minute and then I hear, "Hey buddy! They don't believe it's me. I'm just a little bit dirty from camping out. I was on my way down to the beach house to see you. Can you save us all a trip to the station?"

He puts the arresting officer back on the radio. "Yeah, no doubt about it. That's Steven Mack. What's your twenty? We're on our way to his place now, I can give him a ride home."

He turns the car around and heads back towards the beach. I grin. Nim is fine. Nim sounds happy. We're going to take him home. I'm humming with pleasure.

Sean smiles and winks at me. He reaches for his belt and tosses me a pair of handcuffs. "I can't believe how much you remind me of him, Dave, the older you get. He would never be caught dead riding in a police car unless I let him play with the handcuffs. I'll let you do the honors when we get there."

"Can I keep them, Sean?" I ask excited. I need my own pair for the strip tease act but I really don't want to explain that to him.

"You too? Why am I not surprised?"

When we come around the last bend at the bottom of the mountain there are a half dozen cop cars with lights flashing, but the officers are all leaning against the cars and laughing as the sun goes down. I see Nim covered with dry caked mud except where he's wiped off his face and he's entertaining the crew with some raucous story.

Sean and I get out of the car and Sean shakes his head in amazement. "Rolling in the mud with pigs, Sim? You are definitely going in the back seat!"

"Playing in the river actually," he laughs. "We haven't got a cremation grounds handy to cover myself in ashes, so mud had to do. But I think I've got my divinity back again. It's a dirty job, Sean."

He holds his arms out like a beggar for alms. When I show him the handcuffs he grins and nods. "Bring it on, Dave!" he laughs. "My wife stole my fucking handcuffs. She's going to be punished without mercy."

†

NAT

We sit on the deck all afternoon without talking. She quit crying a long time ago and now she just sits there wearing it, acknowledging the fuck-up and grateful that I'm not preaching to her.

As the sun sets I think I should go home in case Prince needs supervision. Or maybe there's a message. Brandy seems resigned and stable but I don't want to leave her alone here.

It's a long way down from the deck to the forest floor and stronger things than her have been smashed from the fall. I ask her to come back home with me to wait, and she nods and then, as we're leaving, the phone in the bedroom rings.

"Oh," she says flatly. "Nat, for you."

It's Jain and he's jolly, on the verge of tipsy.

"Sweetheart," he purrs, "Can you get in the car and come down here? I want to marry you."

I don't say anything. I wonder if I heard that right.

"Sweet Natasha, it's me and Sim and Dave and Sean and Crystal and we got a license on the Internet. Sean will do it. Come on, baby. If I have to come up and get you I might get arrested."

"Sim? He's okay? He's there with you?"

"Fuck Sim," he laughs. "It's me, Nat. We're having a party; we're not coming home tonight. I want to marry you, baby."

I hear the laughter, uproar and music. "Where?" I ask.

Then Sim gets on the phone and yells, "The beach house, honey. 36th Ave. Make him into an honest man, Nat. We haven't got all night."

And he hangs up on me. But a half minute later the phone rings again. "Don't bring Bran. She's in a whole lot of trouble," he adds then hangs up again.

Ooh. I look at Brandy. I don't want to leave her alone but—wild horses can't stop me.

"Sim's okay," I assure her. "He'll be back tomorrow. But right now I've got to go. I want you to stay with Sunny tonight, okay?" She nods and doesn't object. She's resigned herself to punishment. I take her back to the Ice House and leave her in good hands.

Then I go next door and find Nicky, Prince and Cat playing dice in the boardroom.

"You guys feel like going to a wedding party?" I ask.

†

## JAIN

I'm wrecked. I admit it. But I know this as clearly as water pours on earth. She's coming and I'm marrying her and it's about time. I'm sitting on the beach house deck with Sim, Dave, Sean and Crys. The night sky isn't as crisp here as the mountaintop but we're being compensated by the salty ocean tide. I wonder what it would feel like if you could experience everything at once, Mountain and Sea, Heaven and Earth.

Sim was filthy when we picked him up and he didn't want to go home without getting cleaned up so Sean kept driving down to the sea. Once we got to the beach house he showered and then walked out onto the deck and started inspecting the Universe with Kama Dave. He doesn't seem the least bit interested in leaving.

I'm nearly bouncing off the walls about marrying Nat but Sim and Dave sit like bookends outside. I down a couple of drinks a little too fast, but Crys is the kindest Boddhisatvic bartender in town. She takes my arm and leads me back into the living room and serves me water with lemon and bitters.

"Nice," she says. "Lovely. I love these shotgun weddings, with or without necessity. Love is the drug, Dr. Jain. There's none better."

And I remember her presiding over the party for Sim and Brandy and where did that go? I pray. Oh, I pray Nat will stand by me. I vow to love her and I start cleaning out all the old furniture in my heart to make room for her. As I inspect the bits and pieces I've accumulated, I decide to throw the whole kitchen sink into the ocean and burn the house down for her and start over.

I think of the scar around the back of her heart and how I had the chance to save her life, how she's picked herself back up and how I've taken advantage of her life and her love like the air I breathe. I bite down on my lip and drink some more water. Man, what was that strange sexual stuff she was trying to teach me? Ah. Oh. Ooh. Mm.

I'm humming it. The Ah ruffles my feet and the Mm vibrates my head and then I hear a car pull in and my whole mind dives off the cliff and holds its breath underwater.

Nat, Nicky, Prince and Cat come in the front door and the house comes alive. Nat kisses me and hugs me but then she's right out the back door with Nicky to see the door stop Buddha boys lounging on the deck. My heart sinks a little. A lot. I follow her outside and take a seat on the bare boards of the deck. I may be a doctor and the CEO of Sunrise but I've got a lot to learn about love and the President is a good teacher.

Sim and Dave are meditating and they ignore us so completely that Nat turns back to me and takes my hand. Nicky sits down to meditate with them, cuddling up on Dave's lap and wrapping her legs around him. He doesn't move. I think I learn something about love right then. It doesn't require expression. It doesn't require anything.

So Nat and I, Prince and Cat, Sean and Crys drink a toast in the living room and Sean asks how we want to do this, long or short? I say do it the same way as Sim did it, as few words as possible while still being legal. He laughs, oh I've done many of those.

Prince is understandably nervous. This was his beachfront heroin Quick Stop house not long ago. Now there's a cop living in it. The owner and his junkie landlord are Om'ing on the deck and he's got a beautiful little girl's hand between his knees purring in his ear. He's found himself at the same place but looking on from the other side of the far shore, with an entirely new perspective as a guest.

Eventually Sim comes back into the living room followed by Dave and Nicky. He walks over to Nat and takes both her hands, pulls her to her feet and kisses her pure and sweet like a sister.

But I see love in his eyes and in hers. This is why, I think. This is what stopped me before. If I was jealous of Dave, it's nothing compared to this. How can she love me if she loves Sim? If she loves Dave? I even see her look at Prince like that. How can she love all of us?

Then Sim walks with her and puts her hand in mine and says nothing but he smiles with pure bliss. Sean laughs and says the words and it's done.

†

## S&M

It's chilly and damp when I wake up so I pull her closer to me and bury my face in her neck. Her arms are like soft blankets around me and she smells like roses and saffron. I push my erection hard against her and she laughs.

"S&M? Oh, baby!"

When I open my eyes I'm staring into the sea green eyes of Nicky. She's holding me tight but I can see Kama Dave's arms wrapped around her from behind. We're sleeping like a sandwich on the hard cold deck outside of the beach house. Oh.

Oh!

"Shit, Nick," I groan.

"No," she says. "It's fine. Let me hold you, baby. It's nice to have you back again. Dave doesn't mind."

Dave hums and blinks and laughs.

"Oh, man, the beach house. I fell off the cliff here. It's fricking freezing, Nim. Hold on to us."

He smiles and closes his eyes and then he whispers, "Nicky, maybe you should handcuff him so he can't run away again."

And there I am in the arms of my sweet girl and her husband, my student and practically speaking, my son. My hard-on subsides but I come anyway. It's morning and it never stops.

But the karmic seeds have already been planted in my heart. I've breathed her scent again and tasted her neck and my blood has warmed. Before it gets serious, I pull myself out of Nicky's arms and get up.

Nat married Jain last night and the house is infested with a feast of friends. The bedrooms are full so Prince is curled up on the sofa with the sleeping Cat in his arms. She's got her purple leather pants on but seems to be missing all her clothing above the waist. He's fully dressed but his eyes are open watching her and his cheeks are burning, as red as cherries.

I can't help laughing as I go into the kitchen and boil some water for tea. I'm home again. I'm never leaving here. Fuck Brandy, I think. Rape me once, shame on you. Rape me twice, shame on me. I never want to see that little brown-eyed snake again.

I put some tea leaves in a strainer and pour the boiling water over it and then I watch myself pour the rest of the water all over the back of my hand. Shit. I'm not present; I'm not myself any longer. I see the skin burning before I feel it and then I scream in agony.

Nicky runs into the kitchen and when she sees what I've done, she takes my hand and holds it under the cool water tap.

"It's not as good as what Nat can do," she says, "but it will hold you until we get you home."

"I'm already home," I say. "I'm not going back up there."

She stares at me and then hands me my cup of tea.

"Come and sit down," she says. "Warm up. Are you crazy?"

"Yeah," I say following her into the living room. "Maybe. Probably. I'm over it, Nick. I'm going surfing."

"I'll go with you, beautiful, but don't leave us. Let's just wash out the space between your ears with salt water and see if you don't feel better."

"No, Nick. I'm finished. There's no one up there who needs me. I'm just finished with Sunrise."

I look up and see Dave standing in the doorway, staring at us. He's got four more months of mandatory house arrest. The only reason he's down here is because he's in Sean's custody.

Nat comes out of the bedroom rubbing her eyes and Nicky asks her to take a look at my hand. She hasn't got the oils she needs to treat a burn here and wants to get me home immediately.

"The sooner I can treat it, the better," she advises.

I look in her eyes and remember the promises I made to help her with her own injuries. What kind of boss have I been? I know exactly what she needs to do to get the range of motion back in her lats and keep the scar tissue from permanently disabling her.

But my anger is burning in my stomach and my pride is pulsing in my throat. What kind of husband have I been? I don't want to face my failure.

"No," I say. "I'm going to move back down here with Sean and Crystal. I'm never going back. Have Sage deliver some oils here."

"Then I'm not going back either," Nat says, "I work for you. I'll quit."

"You just married Jain. He bought the damn house," I swear. "Are you going to leave him up there alone with Dave and Nicky?"

"What about my job, Sim?" Prince whimpers. "Do you still need a chef if you're going to live down here?

And suddenly I hear a horrible sound rising in the room. I look up and see Dave muffling the noise with his fist in his mouth and he's crying like a baby.

"Ah, shut up!" Prince moans. Cat wakes up and realizes her semi-nakedness, sits up tall and smiles with pride. It doesn't seem to bother her to be topless in a room with three men. And then there're five men as Jain and Sean come out to see what all the noise is about.

Instead of comforting Dave, Nick turns her glowing eyes on me and hisses with her hard limit, no compromise, take-no-prisoners tone of voice.

"S&M," she demands. "You are coming with me. Now."

She taps her fingernail on my arm and then digs all four fingernails into my skin like little knives.

"Come," she says.

I get to my feet. "Yes, Nicky," I say. "I'm coming with you."

†

SEAN

Nat sits up front with me on the way up the mountain. I've got the lights and siren going because she says the burn is serious enough that time matters.

Sim and Dave are in the back seat with Nicky in the middle.

"How about the handcuffs, Nim?" Dave offers. "Don't you want to wear them in the car? I've got my own now."

"Fuck off," Sim growls. "I'm not in the mood for games at the moment.

"Oooh, Dave," Nicky purrs. "When did you get those? Let me play with them."

I hear a lot of giggling and swearing, pushing and shoving, and Sim raises his voice, "I'm warning you. Leave me the fuck alone. Get your hands off—"

"Behave," Nicky commands him and everything goes quiet in the back seat for a few minutes.

"Brandy will be relieved to see you, boss," Nat says turning around to look in the back seat and then she starts and puts her eyes back on the road.

I look in the rear view mirror and see that Nicky's got one arm around each of their shoulders She's got Sim's left wrist handcuffed to Dave's right wrist on her lap. I crane for a second look and see Sim's head against her neck with his eyes closed. Dave is grinning at me in the mirror.

I start laughing and Nat gives me a worried look.

"Don't worry about it, Nat," I say. "They've been fooling around with each other for six years now. It's just a game. They look pretty, uh—contained don't you think?"

We're almost home and Nat's lost in her thoughts when Nicky says, "Hey, Nat. What are you going to hit him with when we get home?"

"What?!" Nat jumps. "I'm never going to hit him again. It's not my job!"

Sim snorts and opens his eyes and grins.

"I think she means, what kind of medicine are you going to hit me with, honey."

"Oh, that. We've already got the best stuff in the lab. The same extracts I use on yours scars are wonderful for burns. French lavender and helicrysum. And we've got lots of it."

"Nice," he says. Then he adds, "I bet you'd hit me again if I asked very nicely."

She turns around and stares at him. Either she realizes he's teasing or she decides to play.

"Sure," she says. "Especially now that you've disturbed my honeymoon. I think something could be arranged if you begged."

We pull into the driveway and I have to deal with the back seat crew getting unlocked and untangled before they can get out of the car. I'm just happy to get rid of them so I can drive back down the mountain to the real world.

†

NAT

Sim follows me into the lab and I put the helicrysum and lavender on his burn, neat—full strength. He's sullen and disconsolate. When I ask him what happened he just says he poured boiling water on himself.

"I just did it," he observes coolly.

"You're unglued, boss. You can use some grounding. Let me do the rest of your body with something calming."

He shrugs and undresses and gets on the table.

"Nice way to spend your honeymoon," he observes. "Just don't talk to me, okay? I don't want a lecture."

"Brandy tried to hurt herself too yesterday," I offer. "I sat with her all day, but Nicky was really hard on her."

"I said I don't want to talk about it, Nat," he hisses.

"Okay, but you've only been married three months and it takes some time to sort a marriage out. She's very sorry—"

"Not as sorry as she's going to be," he growls and jumps off the table with only one arm oiled, pulls his sweat pants on and slams the door on his way out.

†

## JAIN

When Prince and I get home, Sim is drinking bourbon with Dave in the boardroom, just shutting down. I go into the lab to let Nat know I'm home and she looks really depressed.

"I've just got to take care of some board business with Mack. He called me on the way home. But after that, I'm all yours, sweetheart. I promise. Give me an hour, okay?"

She nods sadly and barely returns my kiss. Strange start to a honeymoon. I thought everything would be cool once we found Sim, but apparently the drama isn't over.

"Why are you mad at us, Nim?" Dave is whining when I return. "Don't leave us like that. The whole place was worried. I didn't like it."

"It's not you, Dave. It's Brandy. She was very bad and I had to take some time out."

"What happens now?" he continues. "Are you going to throw all the furniture off the deck again? She's a good girl. You should keep her. She took care of me when I was sick. And I wanted – "

"You wanted a mother? Tough. You've already got my girl friend. Brandy's fucked up, Dave. I don't want to see her again."

"Did she break your heart?" Dave asks. "You said there's nothing you can do wrong with love."

"I said love, not lust. You know the difference."

"Sorry to interrupt," I say cautiously. "Mack just called a board meeting and wants to see us in the office."

"What can't wait a day so you can have a honeymoon, Jain?" Sim complains.

"I have no clue, Sim. Mack called me on the way home. He probably just wants to make sure you're okay."

When we get to the Fire House, the office door is open and Mack is sitting with Brandy. Sim stops in his tracks at the door and swears.

"I don't want to see her, Mack. Either she leaves or I do."

Mack puts his hand on hers and whispers something and she gets up quickly staring at Sim like a pitiful beggar. He won't even look at her and shuts the door behind her quietly.

"What's the order of business?" he barks. "Because the President usually sets the agenda."

"Staff," Mack says.

"Oh, good then. I want to talk about staff. Fire her, Mack."

"Hey, slow down, brother," Mack warns. "I want to talk about the APB. You were gone for two days without giving any notice or telling anyone. Why shouldn't we fire you?"

"Drugs, brother. She shot me up and fucked me over. I was so whacked I didn't know what I was doing. That's assault. That's against our prescription drug abuse policy. Fire her. Or didn't she tell you about that?"

Mack stares and shakes his head. "No. She said you had a fight. Can I get her back in here and ask about it?"

"As long as I don't have to talk to her, fine," he says.

"The silent treatment, Steven?" Mack wonders.

"For starters," he hisses. "Maybe murder will come next if you don't get rid of her. Keep her away from me, brother."

He picks up the phone and she comes back in cautiously a few minutes later. Mack asks her to sit. She's Sim's wife, but Mack is her boss.

"Did you give him any drugs, Brandy? Anything unauthorized?"

"Yes," she whispers. "It was a horrible mistake. I didn't think—I" She stops and sobs. "I'm sorry, Sim. I should be punished. What can I do?"

"Shit, Sim," I intervene. "You forgave me for beating up on Dave. He even forgave me. Why don't you give her another chance?"

"You were in pain," she pleads. "I thought it would help."

"That's not why she did it, Mack," he hisses. "It was fucking date rape. She knew what she was doing."

Mack considers it with a frown and then says, "But you're married."

"Not for long," he threatens and Brandy starts bawling.

"Please, Sim! Sometimes you're patient with me but sometimes you just tease me. I never know. Sometimes you like to go hard and kinky. Sometimes you don't. I don't understand you. Please. Teach me. What do you want?"

"Look," Mack says, trying to be fair. "You're not the easiest guy in the world to get along with, Steven. To be fair to her, she didn't know what she was getting into when she married you. It was your idea and you insisted on doing it.

"What if I just put her on probation for a week, keep her here in the nurses' room under house arrest and let you think things over? I don't want to lose her. Maybe you'll reconsider.

"I don't know who abused who, but I'm guessing the only harm is to your pride, Steven. How many women have you taken advantage of?

This might be a little karmic consequence coming back to bite you. What do you think?"

"Fuck off, Mack, is what I think," he swears and storms out of the office, headed back to the forest.

"Let him cool off, Brandy," Mack consoles her. "You're under house arrest for a week. If you've got any more drugs, let Sunny know so she can lock them up in the pharmacy. Welcome back to the Ice House."

I've been married less than 24 hours now and I'm starting to wonder what I've gotten myself into.

†

DJ

It has to be done. Nim's heart is broken but it's nothing we can't fix. He has fixed us so many times and we love him. I tell Nick what I want to do and she smiles her beautiful loving smile.

"I agree, baby Dave," she purrs. "It has to be done."

Jain comes back to the Fire House and swears, "Fucking bad day to get married I guess."

But Nicky soothes him and says we will fix everything. We'll stay out of the house so you can have some peace with Nat. What you do with Prince is up to you but he's going to have the rock music on so loud, it won't matter.

We go over to the pool house to find Nim but there's no one there. The bed is unmade and his new leathers are draped over a chair. Nick taps her finger on the mirror.

"Take a good look, Kamadev," she says softly. "There is the God of Love looking back at you. S&M

used to come just looking at his own reflection. I think he sees himself in you."

"What's it mean, Nicky?" I wonder.

"I haven't got a clue, baby," she laughs. "I thought maybe you could tell me. He likes to see you happy. He loves you. Has he ever kissed you?"

"Silly Nicky, he's smacked me once or twice as a joke. He said he doesn't want to make a habit of it. He'd rather fight me. I'm pretty sure he'd rather kiss *you*. Would you kiss him and make it all better?"

"I've never kissed him properly, but I bet I could—if you asked me nicely."

"Nick," I beg her, "we should adopt him. I wanted him to adopt me but now I think we need to take care of him. He's very disturbed."

"Adopt him? How?"

"As your boyfriend. I want to adopt him as your boyfriend. His heart is broken and we love him, Nicky. We can take care of him if Brandy doesn't. You know how."

Her eyes burn. She knows exactly how. Her mouth spreads into the most beautiful heart-stopping man-killer smile. She is the most divine goddess on the planet and she belongs to me. She's much better than a pair of handcuffs if I want to keep Nim.

"You're the most beautiful twisted little fuck in the universe, Kamadev," she sighs.

I laugh. I know I am. I'm the God of Love and Nim taught me everything he knows. I'm going to shoot him so full of sex arrows he won't know what hit him.

†

## S&M

When I come back up the forest trail, I see lights on in my house and I'm furious because Brandy is supposed to be barred. I bang the front door open and see Nicky and Dave sitting on my bed.

"What? Fucking what now?" I growl.

They don't say a word. Nicky just looks at me with that dominatrix stare and Dave looks at me like a lost boy. I'm powerless. I'm fucked.

What? What I wonder? I suck the air in and blow it back out. My planet has been raped and pillaged. I don't speak the same language any more as the happily ever after married couples.

"Go home," I snarl at them. "Fuck off. Get back to the Fire House with the newlyweds, back to the burning house of love with Nat and Jain. Nice job and about time for them, but I'm over it. I'm giving up sex again."

"Nim," Dave whines, "We want to take care of you."

"Yeah, right. Fuck off. Psycho Dave."

Nicky stands up and puts a finger on my heart and snarls, "You. Listen."

"What?"

"We have a proposition for you. Fuck the Fire House. Let's burn *your* house down."

"Uh? Huh?" I stammer.

Dave pulls a chair up and sits on it backwards straddling it.

"Do you want to play?" he smirks. "We know some really nice stuff, Nim."

Nicky walks around behind Dave and starts toying with his leather belt, untying it but not pulling it out, teasing me with her eyes. Oh, I remember this stuff; I remember her doing the same things to me. Nice way to burn off sexual tension. But they're amateurs, both of them. I'm bleeding to death.

"Ask me," Dave says.

"What?" I groan. "Ask you what?"

"Ask me nicely," he says.

And then it hits me. It's not a tease. It's real. I know the game. I consider whether I want to play. His smirk. Her smile. My pain. My best friends. I die a thousand times and my blood starts to boil.

"Can I play please?" I grovel.

Dave grins enormously but Nicky frowns.

"I don't think he sounds serious, baby," she scolds. "Maybe he would be more convincing on his knees."

"Nim. Ask her nicely," Dave insists.

I'm hurt. The pain from my hand radiates in agony inwards from my skin and my wife's betrayal radiates outward from my heart. Where they meet a tidal wave of humiliation and despair crests over me. I don't care anymore that Dave is here or if he sees me like this now.

I sink down on my knees and bow my head to her.

"Nick. Play me. I'm begging you."

Dave pulls the braided leather fringe belt out laughing and holds it out to her, but he doesn't give her the reins. He's driving; I'm amazed and shocked.

"Put your hands on the back of the chair, Nim," he instructs. "Just pretend there are handcuffs because we haven't got any handy. Your fucking wife stole yours," he teases.

I do exactly what psychotic Kamadev tells me to do. I wish he had a loaded gun pointed at my heart. I wish he'd finish me off.

"Nick," he commands, "make it better."

And this surprises me because she doesn't hit me, she leans down, pulls my head back by my hair and French kisses me. She's never in six years kissed me with more passion than a mother or a sister but now she lays it all on me as thick as honey. And only then, when I'm helplessly melted, she takes his belt and hits me. Hard. Intentional. Disciplined.

Kamadev watches amused. His arrows have pierced my heart. I could kill him.

"You fucking pervert, Dave," I swear. "I really don't need any more sexual abuse today."

"Nim," he commands, "we're going to take care of you. We've agreed. There are two of us and only one of you. You will not throw the furniture off the deck. You will not hurt yourself. There's nothing wrong with your heart that we can't fix."

He pulls me up to my feet and puts his palm flat on my chest. I feel an ocean of prana rolling into me. He knows stuff. Shit, I taught him, Nicky taught him, Nat taught him, and apparently he just guessed the rest. He knows more than I do now.

"I think you better leave, the sooner the better," I hiss.

"Can't do that, S&M," Nicky purrs. "We promised Jain and Nat we'd give them a little privacy.

"What about my privacy?"

"We don't think it's good for you right now, baby. Consider yourself our prisoner."

She pulls me away from Dave and puts her arms around me with her hands on my back, one behind my waist and one behind my heart.

"You know I've always respected your celibacy, baby, but you gave it up when you married that nurse. We promise not to abuse you. And I absolutely promise not to try anything straight," she laughs. "But I don't want to hit you anymore."

She kisses me again with the heat of an atom bomb and puts one of her hands on my cock. "Baby, I have always wanted this, you fucking tease," she moans.

"Fuck, Dave," I swear, "Control your wife. This is so wrong!"

Dave laughs and says, "I *am* controlling her. There's nothing wrong with any kind of sex if it's done with love and devotion. You said so yourself, Nim. We love you. Let us in."

"Us? Fuck!"

Dave casually strips off his leathers and climbs into my bed.

"Remember the rules of Shiva dice, Nim," he laughs. "The Universe doesn't like everything to be even. Odd pairs are much more interesting."

Nicky pulls my sweat pants down and kisses me where no married woman belongs. I nearly have a heart attack as she pulls her dress off but I'm so shattered and overheated now I can't stop any of it.

"It's not lust, baby," she says. "It's only love. We want to keep you safe and warm. We don't want you to hurt yourself."

She pulls me into bed and backs up against Dave while she holds me close. He wraps his arms around her as she kisses me. I watch him watching me eagerly and then she turns her back on me and kisses him. So I hold her and watch. Things are getting complicated.

There's enough of her to go around. I hold her while she holds him and then she turns back to me again. I remember she said dream sex goes all night; it never ends. Tantric sex never finishes. It drove Brandy crazy but it's what I love the best.

I don't care about anything else now. I cry with happiness when she takes me inside her and just holds me without moving, completely in control. Then she gives Kamadev a turn. She smells like roses and saffron and feels as soft as silk. She tastes like cinnamon and sugar and sounds like a big cat purring.

When I close my eyes I leave my body, and when I open them again I see Kamadev's approval and love. My God, doesn't the boy have any jealousy? Nicky's green eyes are glazed with ecstasy behind half closed eyelids as she fucks me while he kisses her neck.

"Don't leave us again, Nim," Dave commands. "I'm adopting you as my wife's boyfriend. You make her very happy."

I can see I do. Her happiness makes him a very happy man. And I can't remember ever feeling happier, safer, more loved and cherished in my life than I do now. When she turns again to fuck her psychotic husband, I take my turn worshipping her neck. Kamadev smiles in rapture and winks at me.

Sometime during the night I fall into deep healing dreams but then she wakes me up again with gentle kisses. Dave snorts a little in his sleep and then she falls asleep with me inside her. The next time I wake he's pulling her off me and laughing and then I dream again.

I'm floating on the back of a serpent in a lake of milk, covered with a blanket of jasmine and rose petals. A crescent moon is disappearing on the horizon and the black night is studded with shooting stars.

I dream I'm pouring milk all over the back of my hand while my wife pours some on my cock and rubs it with honey as she kisses it again. The milk pours off my body down into the forest and fills the stream with sticky white jasmine blossoms.

By morning all my pain and betrayal have been snuffed. I'll never be celibate again. I don't feel raped anymore; I feel loved. Nicky is snoring softly as the dawn starts to fill the room with light but Dave's eyes are wide open and dancing with delight, like a boy who's shared his most precious toy and discovered how to really play.

"My god, Kamadev," I whisper. "How do you two ever manage to get out of bed?"

"Pancakes, Nim," he grins. "Thank goodness you hired Prince for us or we wouldn't know when to stop."

†

NICK

"Nim hasn't got a bath, Nicky," Dave explains, "but there's a huge shower. Come on."

I follow him into the bathroom and it's already steaming with hot vapors and sandalwood oil. When I step into the shower, S&M pulls me against him and oils my back. He's lost all his reserve and his hard boundaries and smiles as sweetly as a pet, our newly adopted stray wild animal.

When we're all clean and well anointed, S&M picks up his leathers and looks at them like a stranger and smiles.

"Experienced beyond your years, Kamadev," he laughs. "How did you know I needed these? I need them now more than pancakes."

He wriggles into them and they're almost too tight since they're so new, but they'll relax with time and mellow just as he has. He admires himself in the mirror and ties his belt around his hips half in the loops and half hanging loose. He looks deadly dangerous and I'm already thinking of taking them off him again.

"Nicky," Dave commands, "behave. It's time for breakfast."

"I've got a proposition now," S&M smiles, "after breakfast. I haven't got a bathtub but there's a beautiful stream down in the woods where we can soak and meditate. I spent all day in the water. We can just disappear there."

I'm grateful he wants to spend more time with us instead of running away again. We walk back to the Fire House for breakfast together, arms wrapped shamelessly around each other's waists.

Walking between these beautiful half naked men is just as erotic as sleeping between them. My love for Kama Dave is only magnified by my love for S&M and I'm intoxicated with bliss.

Prince is waiting patiently in the kitchen with his pancake batter and sweet apple sauté. Jain and Nat are still in bed and no one's shown up for breakfast. He looks at us sheepishly, happy to have customers but a little confused, so I just take him in my arms and kiss him like he's never been kissed. Even that little Cat Girl can't kiss like I do.

I take him beyond shock into awe and when I let him go, he's got a smile bright enough to restore sight to the blind. Dave laughs but warns, "Don't make a habit of it, Nicky. You're only allowed to kiss our prisoners."

## Part Two: LEATHER AND LACE

***"Mother flies mind kites in the winds of hope
held by the strings of maya.
Of a hundred thousand only one or two break
free
and you Mother laugh and clap your hands."***
**~ Ramprasad**

# Part Two: Leather and Lace

†

## JAIN

"Rick," Nat whispers, "I want to show you something new, something a little different."

She started calling me by my first name the night before last when we were married. I like the sound of it. No one ever calls me that. Everyone else uses either Jain or Doctor Jain. Except for Sim, when he gets really cocky, who likes to call me Lover Boy because he set me up with her and I was as easy as pie.

I should have married her three months ago when she started sleeping with me, but I guess I was a little nervous. She knows a lot of sexual stuff and I was jealous of how close she is to all the other men—and boys—in the house.

I'm just a little nervous again, but she says it's not going to be sex right now; it's another kind of pleasure, some Tantric yoga.

"Trust me, Rick," she says. "You married a Tantrika. You might as well enjoy all the fringe benefits. It's not sex but it improves the health of your entire sexual system."

I remember Kamadev said she taught him kundalini Tantra so I ask if this is how she did it. She laughs and says no, she's been saving it for me. She puts some pillows under my knees and tells me to relax and behave. And then she sits on my right side and puts her left hand on my heart and her right hand between my legs.

But it's not where she usually puts her hand. She doesn't touch my cock; she massages right behind my balls, the pelvic floor, the perineum. I'm a doctor, so I know these things. What the fuck though? It's actually more relaxing than erotic.

"Nat? Honey, what are you doing?" I ask confused.

"Just taking care of your first chakra, baby," she explains. "The nerves running to all of your sexual apparatus run through the perineum. This refreshes, relaxes and helps to rejuvenate all your sexual nerves.

"When your nerves are relaxed your body feels better and functions better. It's very good for your sexual health. Be still. I'm going to take very good care of you, Doctor."

She takes her time and he's right as usual. I feel like I'm floating. Then she moves her right hand and cups my sex organs and holds me quietly. She doesn't stroke me sexually; she just holds me for a few minutes.

"The same chakras that exist in you spine also exist on a concentrated level in your penis, from the root to the crown," she continues.

"Very powerful stuff you guys have to deal with perpetually, two mirrors of pranic energy. I'm jealous on one level but relieved on another that I don't have to be a pranic schizophrenic with energy going in two directions simultaneously."

I feel my heart beating slower as the tension in my muscles dissolves. The beautiful scents of breakfast waft into the bedroom and then I hear a sound I've never heard before: Prince laughing like a maniac.

"To be continued," she promises. "I can show you some more after breakfast. Maybe we should check on them, Rick," she laughs. "Just to be sure they're not burning the house down."

The boardroom table is half covered with cold breakfast plates. Prince, Sim, Nicky and Dave are all huddled around the other end over Dave's giant Monet lily pond puzzle.

Sim winks at me and Dave gets up like a gentleman to pull a chair out for Nat. It looks like they're contained, but all their eyes are burning with glee. I marvel at how Sim has turned from a raging train wreck to blissful peace so quickly.

I sit with Nat at the business end of the table and pour us some coffee. When I look up I see amused excitement in her eyes too.

"One more piece!" Prince begs, holding up a finger. "Then I'll make a fresh batch of pancakes for you."

"Okay, honey," she tells him. "Take your time."

She looks at me again with a raised eyebrow and I take another look at the players. While Prince has his head down diligently searching for a home for his puzzle piece, the rest of them are passing red-hot smoldering smiles around their end of the table.

Sim is winking at Nicky, then grinning at Dave. Nicky is smirking at Dave and snarling at Sim. The smiles between Sim and Kama Dave are profoundly disturbing.

I give myself a second reconsidered opinion. The house *is* burning down. Sim catches my eye and laughs contentedly.

"We've got a very special wedding present for you, Jain," he says. "Nicky and I are taking Dave for a little excursion this afternoon. Prince will be serving you a private dinner here tonight. Don't wait up for us. We've got things going on, Lover Boy."

Prince places his puzzle piece and howls again with joy, then jumps up to make more breakfast. As soon as he's out of the room, the scorching smiles and eye play intensify. Nicky puts her head on Sim's shoulder and Dave snorts with joy.

"Steven," I interrupt, "What the fuck is up with you guys?"

"Everything, Jain," he laughs. "Anything and everything. Is there a problem?"

Nat smiles sweetly and says, "Not for me, boss. I never want to see you as low as you were yesterday. It's good to see the leathers back and the smack in your face attitude.

"Don't you think he looks happy, Rick?" she continues, turning to me.

"Uh, I'm not sure, baby. He looks like a time bomb from where I'm sitting. He looks like a maniac. Are you okay, Steven?"

"Never better," he smirks and points out a puzzle hole for Dave's piece. "That's what I'm talking about," he grunts. "Even better than these water lilies. It's going to kill you, honey. Just wait until you see it."

In a little while Prince comes back with plates of omelettes, pancakes and spicy apples and sets them proudly in front of us.

"Eat your breakfast, Rick," Sim says, amusing himself with my first name. "You need your strength. You probably have enough of your own sex life to concentrate on without worrying about mine."

Prince goes back into the kitchen and returns with a big picnic basket and Sim gets up and hands him a little stack of hundred dollar bills.

"Take Sunny shopping with you too so you can buy some nice champagne. Keep the change."

"Thanks, boss!" Prince laughs and pockets the money. "Have fun with the picnic."

When he leaves the room again, Nicky stands up behind Sim and puts both her hands on his hips, cuddling up to his backside. Dave gets up and smacks her on the ass.

"Behave, Nicky," he scolds with a laugh. "Not in public."

"Ooooh, Baby Dave," she purrs. "Then why don't we go somewhere more private?" She picks up the picnic basket and leads the way out of the house.

I'm not sure if we're being treated to a wedding dinner or simply bribed.

"Don't worry, Rick," Nat smiles. "They'll be fine. They're just good friends."

"Right. Friends. But I've got a sinking feeling, Mrs. Jain, that someone is going to get hurt. Hurt very badly."

†

## PRINCE ALBERT

S&M gave me $500 to cook a private wedding dinner for Dr. and Mrs. Jain. I like calling her Mrs. Jain now because she blushes so sweetly when she hears it.

That's $500 on top of the already generous salary he pays me monthly and I'm grinning with pride. I remember the first time I met him when he split my head open for dealing dope and robbed me of $800. It's a lot better being on his side.

I offer to make anything their hearts desire but Nat just says, "Surprise us, honey."

I think hard about it and decide to start them off with oysters topped with lime granita and a sprinkle of caviar, rose champagne, a salad with baby lettuce, goat cheese and toasted almonds.

I don't want to be too cheap and keep too much for a tip but I have to think hard to even spend three or four hundred dollars on ingredients for dinner for two.

So I think of chateaubriand with béarnaise sauce, herb roasted new potatoes, young asparagus and the most wicked old Cabernet Sauvignon I can find. I can get the tarragon, chives, rosemary and thyme fresh from Brandy's garden, much nicer than anything I would find at the market.

For dessert, I'll make the most difficult thing I know, a Grand Marnier soufflé served with cut cane Semillon. I start to wonder if $500 will cover all that, but I don't care anymore about the tip. I've got all day to shop and cook and there's nothing I would rather do.

"Don't forget to feed yourself too, Chef," Nat teases and my mouth is already starting to water.

I go over to Mack's house to get Sunny since I'm too young to buy alcohol and I find her sitting in the kitchen with Brandy. Brandy has a very sad face, but she looks happy to see me and gives me a sweet kiss on the cheek.

"I miss everyone already," she moans. "I've got six more days locked up here and then I don't want to think about what will happen to me after that."

I don't think anyone is actually missing her in the least, but I don't want to hurt her, so I change the subject and ask if I can get some of the herbs from her garden on the deck behind the pool house.

"Of course you can. Isn't Sim home?"

"I don't think so," I mutter. "I think he's off meditating somewhere."

"He's gone again? I hope he's okay. If the house is locked I can give you a key. I'm not allowed over there now."

She sighs and stares at the wall. I see tears starting so I tell Sunny she's supposed to take me shopping. Now.

†

## S&M

Nick is off the charts with joy as we start down the forest trail. It's complicated. It's nice, but at the same time I'm a little delirious with the whole situation. At least they don't work for me, but they're my patients and my students. We're all close friends but now we've gone across the line of friendship into intimacy.

On one hand, a yoga teacher isn't supposed to sleep with students. But who is teaching whom now? The lines are crisscrossing and tangled. On the other hand, Shiva slept with his first yoga student, his wife Parvati. But I've feel like I've failed terribly for not being able to teach my wife what I wanted her to know.

How could I? All I really knew about transcendental sex was how to control my own kundalini energy, how to have endless orgasms by meditating. I start wondering if that was just pranic masturbation. How would I know?

Seven years of celibacy has really messed me up. Sure, I've got control, but it's ruined me for straight sex and I—hell, I've got to think about this.

What I did with Nicky and Dave all night was something I've never done before. Not like that. That sex hit all my koshas at once: physical, pranic, mental, emotional and spiritual. It stunned me with its pure power.

What did Nat tell me? Kamadev refined and redefined transcendental sex. He took what she taught him and ignited it with pure unconditional love.

They just raised the bar of passion and desire. Rajas and Vasana. Shit. I'm supposed to be going in the other direction. My inner peace has been shot full of love oils and flower-decked arrows and the sweet seductive smiles of my friends.

I'm not talking to them now. I'm speechless. All the way down to the stream I'm leading the way just mulling, nodding, pointing, laughing, thinking, listening to their delight. I'm wondering who the fuck taught Nicky how to do that? It surely wasn't me. It was Kamadev, the transcendental sexual master. And who taught him? He was a psycho junkie virgin a couple of months ago—until he got lessons from the Tantrika herself, Nat.

Who's going to teach me how to teach my wife what I don't really know? Dave? Nicky? Nat? Who's got me? The more I think about it, the more confusing it becomes.

No wonder Brandy lost control with me. I showed her Tantra and rough stuff and loving things and straight sex but it was never the same twice. She said I confused her, that I was too wild. And all along I was just making it up, trying to teach her something I've imagined but never done before. But now I've done it and I'm disintegrating.

No wonder Shiva was celibate for a thousand years. It's complicated. Marriage, fuck! Maybe I should go back to being the town slut. Nah, that's too easy. It was fun when I was 18 but it didn't work out very well.

I try to turn my mind off and be present in the forest but it's like trying to keep a monkey still by holding its tail.

I lead them down the little cut off from the trail straight through the bush and have to concentrate a little harder on where I'm going. I bring my thoughts back to my breath and to the feel of the forest floor on my bare feet.

And then I hear the murmuring of the stream below as the water polishes the rocks and stones with infinite care and I quit worrying about sex and marriage and propriety and ignorance and failure. I can't understand any of it—yet. How would I know?

As soon as the little river comes into view, Kama Dave howls like a puppy. He's nearly whimpering as he strips naked.

"Oh, man Nim!" But I'm way ahead of him. I knew what was coming.

There are pools with water lilies floating on the surface fringed with horsetail grass and narrow torrential currents where the water gushes passed rock piles. Flowering vines drip from low hanging branches overhead and fallen blossoms drift into the still pockets of the river.

The forest scent is an intoxicating woody blend of fir, pine, juniper and spruce with overtones of jasmine and honeysuckle. I wade into the icy cold water and find a deep spot wrapped and tangled in water lilies and sit on the muddy river floor. The water is black as night in the shadowy pools and crystal clear where it spurts and gurgles around the rocks.

I inhale my beautiful Divine Mother's scent. This is my girl. This is my soul, my love. It's in me and all around me. It's the river and the forest and the air I breathe and the sound of Dave snorting with shock as he steps into the cold current.

I exhale everything that ever hurt me and start laughing like a madman, watching Dave watching Nicky step out of her dress. I don't care about lines anymore.

†

## NAT

It's not like I need to improve the beautiful doctor's performance. Since he quit using steroids, I've got no complaints. But he has no idea how much further we can take this, and I want him to help me teach. I love him just as he is, a man; but with that extraordinary body and heart and mind, he could easily become a god.

The world is endless divine perfection but it can never have enough divine personifications as far as I'm concerned. I want to take Rick where Kamadev's gone. I want to take Sim there too. I'm surprised Sim is so sexually confused for a Tantric yogi but Mother Nature doesn't approve of a celibate Sex God and has cursed him accordingly with a little perversion—okay maybe a lot.

Brandy said he's too wild and maybe he's too strong, too tough to be receptive. I know his highest intention is strength on every level. I want to wake up the man's divine femininity. Strength doesn't have to be cruel and hard.

Brandy wanted to soften him up and so do I, but she hasn't a clue how to do it. Drugs, hah! So harsh and hard. Rape, so brutal. It's not submission that Nature wants; it's union, yoga.

I know this stuff. And what better man to practice it on than my new husband, straight, hard and beautiful? It's my dharma as a Tantrika to pour cool compassion on the fires of desire, to elevate beings above suffering.

I clear the breakfast plates so Prince can go shopping and while I wash the dishes I can feel my husband watching me in all the colorful shades of curious.

†

DJ

Nim is so happy now soaking in the little river and singing bursts of dirty blues, but he's not talking much. I can see the wheels in his head turning. Nicky wants to tease him and play some sexy games with him but I pull her away and tell her not to hassle Nim now. He's very calm and not to be disturbed I tell her. So let him be.

I don't even let her kiss me. I don't want to steam the peaceful forest up with passion right now. I just want to relax and play and maybe nap since we've been up all night. She keeps begging me for kisses and I just say keep it up, Nicky. I love to hear you beg like that.

I pin her arms to her side and make her sit quietly in the water and be a good girl. When Nim finally stands up and climbs back up the bank of the river to dry off in the sun, I let her go with clear firm instructions to behave and serve our picnic lunch.

She makes a face at me and scrunches up her nose and turns her green eyes on me trying to melt my heart, but I command her with a steel blue serious stare. It works.

"Oh yes, Master," she smiles submissively. "I'm your prisoner."

She gets the picnic basket and spreads out a table cloth on the grassy bank and sets out the containers and plates, fruit, cheese, deviled eggs, sour dough bread, nuts, olives and sangria, a beautiful little feast. I sit next to her just as she opens the last container with some pieces of carrot cake. She laughs, breaks off a piece and stuffs it into my mouth.

And then she wins. I know I'll never control her unless she wants to play. I love her too much.

"Come, S&M," she orders him. "Don't keep us waiting."

She picks up the white blessing scarf from the heap of clothing and I think she's going to put it around my shoulders but she surprises me. Instead, she wraps it across my eyes and ties it behind my head in a blindfold.

"Now, Master, I'm going to feed you. Just tell me what you'd like," she laughs.

"Cheese," I say and I open my mouth for it. But what she puts in my mouth is a couple juicy grapes. I like the surprise. It's a good game and I bite into them and laugh.

"Cake," I try next and I get a nice bite of creamy deviled egg.

I hear Nim snickering and helping himself to a plateful of food and then he says, "Hey Kamadev, how about a little bit of cheese?" He feeds me some almonds instead.

Nicky takes my hand and puts a glass in it and says "You need to drink your milk, baby." I put it to my lips and taste the sweet citrus, prosecco and port in the sangria.

And now I don't even bother to tell them what I want, I just open my mouth and take what I get, bits of bread and finally a surprising piece of cheese, some olives, more grapes and nuts and a little bit of Nicky's tongue which she sneaks into my mouth after a bite of cake.

Nim keeps filling my glass and pretty soon I start to feel the nap coming over me. When we've polished off the feast, we all lie down in the shade. I keep the blindfold on so Nicky can't tempt me with those wicked smiles. With her as a pillow between us we snore off into the afternoon without even any sex.

†

## S&M

It takes a little convincing for my jailors to understand it's okay for them to let me go—in fact I really need some time out to think.

"Look, I feel grateful and blessed for all the love and attention you've shared, but I'm your teacher and I know what I'm doing. I promise not to harm anything."

When I get home, I kick back on the bed and study the ceiling. I know this ceiling very well and it works better for me right now than a formal meditation. I don't feel like stripping off my leathers in order to sit comfortably in lotus asana. I feel safe and secure in these pants, protected and not so nakedly vulnerable, a lot safer than my handcuffs were.

The entire day was a meditation; now it's time to simply integrate. The ceiling seems to wait patiently for me but it darkens slowly when the light fades as if it's leaving me behind.

I don't feel guilty about anything I've done and I don't feel attached either, but I have a nagging memory of my sweet girl, lost and neglected. My beautiful students Kamadev and Nicky are happy with and without me now; they don't need my attention.

I feel the shift of energy as the sun sets, as Vata time quiets down and shifts into Kapha time. It must be six o'clock. When I was in intensive care that was my Kapha girl's nursing shift, six to ten, morning and night.

I pick up the phone and let it ring a few times and then I hear her whisper, "Sim? Is that you?"

But I don't want to talk to her. I hang up and make another inspection of the ceiling. When the phone rings a few seconds later I ignore it, trying to be cool. I let it ring twenty times or so and when it stops my heart is pounding in the silence.

I do a couple rounds of nadi shodhona and slow my heartbeat back down with my breath, and then I call her again.

"Sim? I know it's you, baby. I can see caller ID."

Good. So I don't have to talk to her. She knows I'm calling. I just hold the phone and listen to her choppy breathing and I know she can hear my breath soft and steady. I hope she doesn't talk anymore. I don't want to hear it.

She listens. Her breath gets a little quieter and she just listens to nothing, just the sound of my breath through my nose, long easy breaths. How long will she listen I wonder? This is a test. Is she still out of control and desperate? Or can she feel me from where she is, upstairs in another house?

I don't hang up this time. I wait a long time. So does she. I wait forty-five minutes until it's fully dark, just breathing quietly, and then I growl in a low voice, rough and gravelly, "Good night, baby."

That's all I've got for her right now. I hope it helps her sleep.

I strip off the leathers and cover myself in sandalwood oil, then step into a steaming shower to open the pores of my skin and drink it in. When I'm done, I switch to cold water to force my blood deeper into my muscle tissue.

When I'm good and frozen, I walk out onto the yoga deck naked and sit on the futon in padmasana, the lotus position, and start deep rhythmic Breath of Fire, driving my seminal fluids into my blood stream and burning off my toxic thoughts.

I sit out there all night, watching the stars shoot and the moon wander, watching the galaxies spin, letting the night blanket me with peace. I think I hear Nicky and Dave giggling in the distance, but I can't be sure if it's a real sound or just an echo left over from the day down in the forest.

When the sky begins to lighten in the east and fade to grey, when I feel like it's 6am, I get up and put my leathers back on and lie down on my bed.

I pick up the phone again and call.

"Sim?" she answers sleepily.

"Come on, honey," I command her.

"I'm under house arrest," she reminds me. "I'm not allowed out."

"Do it anyway," I say and hang up on her.

She comes in barefoot and I get under the sheet with my pants on and hold the edge of the sheet back for her. She lies down next to me and I just hold her. I listen to her breathing and fall into synch with her rhythm. We don't say a word and soon drift into a dream.

Around 10am I wake up and I give her a chaste kiss. I haven't got any more for her. I don't forgive her and I don't really want to talk to her. It feels nice to hold her again but she's become a stranger.

"Wake up, nurse," I say. "Your shift is over. Get out of here."

She gets up to leave but she turns around at the door and makes a really bad mistake. She looks at me for a long time, drinking me with her sad brown eyes. It hurts me to my soul. When she leaves, I get a pen and paper and start to write.

†

JAIN

This is getting interesting. I'm used to taking the lead so it's amusing to let her drive for a change.

"Just keep your mind open, Rick," she coaxes. "Consider that this is going to be delayed gratification. Delayed but perpetual. We're not going to have sex right now, but what I'm going to teach you is going to make sex better than your wildest dreams."

"Honey," I tease, "you don't how wild my dreams are."

"I'll put money on it," she laughs. "Try me."

"If you're just talking about that Tantric stuff Sim is into, nine thousand orgasms without breathing hard, I don't think it's worth the effort. It really doesn't seem to be working out very well for him. His marriage is on the rocks after only three months."

She smiles and takes my hand and leads me into the lab, not the bedroom. Interesting.

"It could work really well for him," she sighs. "It *should* be working out really well for him. He's got his physiology under control, he knows what he's doing and he's wired correctly for it. He's just missing a little piece of the puzzle."

She puts a clean sheet on the massage table while I undress and when I lie on the table she covers me with another sheet.

"Honey, we're married. Nobody's home," I tease.

"That's not the point, Rick. The purpose is to keep it therapeutic so you'll relax. Down, boy.

"Men need to learn to relax and receive. As a man, your sexual conditioning is focused on achieving goals and performing actions. This is a non-sexual massage to teach you to experience receptive pleasure and expand your sexual abilities.

"You're not supposed to do anything except sink into deeper relaxation and enjoy the pleasure. We're not going anywhere with it.

"But after our private dinner tonight there will be a test. Then you can show me how well it works for you when you take it for a test drive."

"Fair enough," I laugh but she's already got me hard just talking about it. "Sorry," I add when she notices.

"No, that's not a problem. You'll get hard and soft and hard and soft, riding waves of pleasure. It's actually a very desirable and therapeutic part of the experience. The point isn't orgasm. It's exploring the edge between orgasm and ejaculation and learning to separate them.

"When you master that, you'll be able to make love as long as you like, and orgasm over and over without losing any semen. But enough theory, just be still."

She gives me a beautiful full body massage and then she spends some time just putting her hands on my chakras and holding them there and when I'm nearly nodding off with relaxed pleasure and drifting away she puts her hands carefully on my cock through the sheet.

I get hard and then soft but I stay relaxed so she puts her hands under the sheet and continues, massaging me carefully and respectfully, slowing it down when I get hard and then waiting.

The longer she goes, the easier it is for me to enjoy it without reacting, just anticipating what will come later without rushing anywhere. And then I have an easy orgasm, gentle but very nice without losing my erection. The sensation isn't localized in my sex organs; it spreads up my spine and even kicks me in the head. We keep going a few more times and I feel pretty sure I've got the hang of it. I feel nice, relaxed and satisfied without finishing.

She puts her left hand on my heart and holds her right hand still on my cock and breathes with me for five minutes without moving.

"Nice job, Doctor," she laughs. "You don't have a lot of negative sexual conditioning to undo. You're going to be an excellent teacher."

"Uh—what? I'm going to be teaching who what?" I don't want to lose the beautiful high I've got going right now by hearing the answer.

"Your prize student, Doctor Rick, your straight A nursing student. She hasn't got a clue how to deal with a celibate Tantric sex god who has years of abusive sexual relationships to unravel.

"That's the little piece of the puzzle that Sim's missing. He doesn't know how to teach her."

I get up from the table and dress slowly. I feel good. I'm too relaxed to be worried about Sim and don't really care that much about fixing his sexual issues. He doesn't seem too worried about it either;

it's more like he's digging a bigger hole to bury himself by his licentious behavior with Nicky and Dave.

But there's an elephant in the room and I've got to ask her or I'll never be able to relax completely with this.

"Did you teach this to Kama Dave, Nat? Did you teach him how to expand his sexual abilities?"

She takes both of my hands and looks in my eyes so I'm forced to see into her heart and her integrity.

"I only taught him how to control his kundalini energy. I didn't have to teach him what I showed you, how to undo his male sexual conditioning because he didn't have any. He was a virgin, Rick. He didn't know anything.

"Once the kundalini serpent woke up in him he didn't need to correct anything. He knew more than me.

"But Sim spent years behaving terribly. You guys told me the whole story, how he took advantage of every girl in town. He's got an environmental disaster to clean up."

†

## BRANDY

At 10am he asks me to leave. I turn back at the door to look at him and feast my eyes, but I know better than to break the silence. As I walk out of the pool house I can see Dr. Jain lifting weights with Nicky and Dave on the far side of the pool.

I wish I could go over and watch them but I'm not allowed. I wave though and the boys wave back. Nicky freezes and glares at me. I can feel her hatred all the way across the lawn.

Well, there it is. At least she knows I was with him. For all she knows I could have been with him all night long. I breathe a long sigh. If only I had been.

All those nights, all those days, a hundred or so that we've been married, I cherished him. I slept with him. I followed him like a puppy. I wanted much, much more from him than he was willing to give, but I had his heart.

I won't give him up. I'll learn to behave the way he wants me. I won't speak to him unless he asks. I won't touch him unless he wants me. But I find it hard not to look at him. More than anything I miss looking into those deep cold blue eyes. His soul is naked in those icy pools.

I walk past Dr. Mack's office on my way to my room. The door is open and he looks up with a questioning expression.

"I'm sorry I left," I say. "He asked me to come over."

"Oh, well, that's good then," he smiles gently. "Is he softening up at all?"

"Still not talking to me, except 'come on', 'do it', 'go away', but I'll take that. It was nice to see him. It gives me a little bit of hope."

"So you didn't make up, then?"

"Hardly. He slept with me for a couple hours with his clothes on. Any advice for me, brother-in-law? I would move heaven and earth to have him trust me again."

He shakes his head. "I don't know him much better than you, Brandy. I thought I did but he keeps surprising me. I'll help you any way I can but I'm not sure how. But Brandy, no matter what he says, I'm not firing you.

"I'm ready to take some more patients on. Sean's coming up to talk with me tomorrow. There's nothing like helping other people to keep yourself out of the deep end of trouble."

"Thanks, Doc," I smile weakly. "Do you have anything good I can study in the meantime? So I can stay out of the deep end?"

"Good? Medical books, hah! Good enough to put you to sleep," he laughs. "Oh, wait. I've got just the thing you need. It might even help you understand your husband a little better. He loved it. Let's see—it's a tiny little book—here it is. Shankara's 'Viveka Chudamani', the Jewel of Perception.

"Steven loved this one. The underlines are his; I don't like to mark my books up but he was 15 when he read this and I couldn't stop him.

He gives me the little book and I flip through it and see the little teen-ager's comments like happy squeals in the margins. I read one of the underlined passages:

*"The self controlled man is illumined when he enjoys eternal bliss. He is entirely merged in the creator. He knows himself to be the unchangeable reality."*

Tears blur the words on the page and I feel like I'm holding my husband's young soul in my hands. I press the little book to my heart and I can't thank Mack enough, so I throw him a kiss and take it back to my room.

†

NAT

Nicky and Dave don't come home until breakfast. They've got the empty picnic basket and stars in their eyes. I ask them how Sim is doing and they look at each other and laugh.

"Sim who?" Nicky teases. "Oh, S&M! He went home yesterday. He looked pretty happy then. He looked pretty too."

I'm not judging my boss but I feel a little bit relieved that the heat in the house has been turned down a notch. Or at least I think so for a few seconds and then I notice Nicky is staring at Rick like she's never seen him before.

"Doctor," she gushes, "what have you done to yourself?" She glances at Kama Dave and then back at Rick. "You've got that aura thing going on. You're glowing."

He just smiles and takes a little sip from his coffee mug. He's beyond beautiful. He knows things now and she knows he knows. He's not straight anymore and he doesn't miss a bit of it.

"I'm afraid you're on your own for breakfast," I warn them. "After that incredible meal last night, I gave Prince the day off. So it's fruit and yogurt or whatever else you feel like fixing."

"Coffee," Dave says. "I don't want to eat yet. How about chest and arms, Doc? I need a pump."

Dave flexes his biceps and I've got to admit he's coming along nicely. He's nowhere near Rick's league, but I imagine what he'll look like in another few years. He's going to be a heart wrecker. I'm a little worried for Nicky. When Dave is Sim's age, she'll be pushing 40.

When they go out to the gym, I decide to pay my boss a visit. I knock on the pool house door and wait a few minutes. When he opens the door, he doesn't say a word, but he gestures for me to come in.

He's not talking and I respect that. It's a common practice for a yogi to maintain long periods of silence for inner transformation. He takes my hand and leads me out to the yoga deck and pulls one of the mats forward to the edge of the deck in teaching position.

My heart jumps in gratitude. I really need this now. I put my hands together in anjali mudra, the gesture of prayer and respect.

"Namaste, Steven," I say respectfully. "I wanted to thank you for the best meal of my life last night and to see if I could do anything to repay you. But now I'm even deeper in debt for your kindness."

I pull another mat up in front of him and stand in readiness, my hands clasped behind my back, my weight perfectly distributed over the four corners of my feet. He looks at my feet and his eyes flow up my legs, my torso, my neck, and then deep into my eyes.

He starts ujayii breath and I follow him for a few minutes. Then he begins a slow and serene moon salutation, Chandara Namaskar. The steady rhythmic dance of the vinyasa flow opens my body and I feel a welcome relief as blood pours into my ribs and waist, kissing my pain and washing through my injuries.

It reminds me that I should be doing this every day on my own. I know it but I appreciate the reminder. We go through eight rounds on each side, sixteen total, and by the time we finish he has a tranquil smile on his lips. He sits down in lotus position and watches me, then he gestures with one finger on his right nostril to begin nadi shodona.

I listen to his breath and synchronize with him, neither of us actually using our fingers; instead we do the advanced pranic version—easy enough to accomplish with a little concentration—inhaling through the left nostril and exhaling through the right, then inhaling through the right and exhaling through the left.

I remember teaching this to Kamadev sitting right here, months ago yet it was another lifetime. We breathe slower and slower until our breathing nearly stops and then lie down in shavasana, corpse pose, to integrate all the beautiful pranic energy we've awakened.

I close my eyes and feel the twitches in my back, in my ribcage, deep in the scarred tissue where healing is accelerating. I feel gratitude and warmth in my heart and I send it back to him with all my love.

Twenty minutes later I feel him tap my forehead and he takes my hand to help me up again. He puts his hands on my shoulders and gives me a squeeze and a smile.

"Thank you," I murmur. "That was beautiful. I'm going over to check on your wife now. I'll tell her you're well. Do you want me to give her any other message?"

His smile disappears and he walks back into the bedroom. I follow him and he hands me an envelope and then opens the door for me to leave.

Brandy is lying on the bed in the nurses' room reading but she jumps up with joy when she sees me.

"Oh, Nat," she smiles, "I'm so happy to see you! I miss everyone. Sit down."

I sit in the chair by the window in the sunshine and she continues like a faucet turned on full. After spending an hour with Steven in silence, it's amusing, but she hasn't had anyone to talk to.

"I saw him, Nat. He called me last night and then this morning he called again and asked me to see him. I feel so much better now. And Doctor Mack gave me this beautiful little book that was Sim's favorite. It's got sweet notes he'd written all through it when he was young. I'm amazed what a jewel he is, how thoughtful he was even as a teenager. I feel so much closer to him now, like he's here in the room with me."

She pauses for a breath and then she sees the letter in my hand and stops.

"Is that for me?" she asks. I nod and hand it to her. She tears the envelope open and immediately her face turns white with shock. She stares at the letter and seems to read it a hundred times and then she hands it back to me.

It's very short and as pointed as an ice pick in the heart. It hurts me to read it.

*That was goodbye this morning, beautiful girl. I can't see you again. I failed you as a husband and I failed you as a teacher. It hurts too much to look at you.*

*You won't have a problem finding employment with recommendations from Mack and Jain, but you can't stay here. I'll send money.*

*Go away.*

I look at her and expect her to cry but she's beyond that.

"Brandy, I don't know what to say," I try. "I want to help you. I think I can."

"Get me a pen," she whispers desperately.

I find a pen in the desk drawer and she takes it, picks up the letter and gets down on her knees on the floor.

"Nicky said he loves to be begged," she seems to be consoling herself, drawing together her courage. She turns the letter over and starts to write quickly, using the floor as her desk. When she's filled the back of the page she hands it to me.

"Give that to him, please. I beg you, Nat. Is it good?"

I look at the page, line after line, over and over.

*I'm down on my knees begging you please, please, please. I'm down on my knees begging you, beautiful husband, please! Please! Please! I would give my life for you. I'm down on my knees begging. Please! Please! Please!*

Over and over and over, as much begging as the paper can hold. Then she takes it back from me and fills all the leftover white space on the other side of the page where he wrote. Her handwriting gets smaller and smaller as she writes so she can fit more pleas on the page. By the time she hands it back to me there are tears streaming down my cheeks.

"Will you tell him?" she begs. "Will you tell him I'm really on my knees?"

"I'll help you, Brandy," I promise. "Doctor Jain is going to help you, too. Just be patient, sweetheart. Keep reading the book."

I take the letter back to the pool house. When Sim answers the door, I put one hand up with my palm open in the mudra for Ahimsa, the gesture for 'no harm' and the most basic tenet of yoga philosophy.

I hand him the letter and then get on my knees in front of him while he looks at it, turning it over again and again with his mouth open.

"She wrote this on the floor on her knees, Steven. Have mercy on her, please."

He breaks his silence at last and says his favorite word, "Fuck!" he moans.

†

JAIN

Nick and Dave train like wild animals, as if they are trying to bury each other alive with their superior beauty. The atmosphere of narcissistic codependency is thick in the air. Nicky flirts with me steadily while Kama Dave is trying to concentrate on his sets; Dave teases her relentlessly with a domineering stare taken straight from S&M's lady-killer chapbook.

Towards the end of the session I see Brandy coming out of the pool house with a sweet wave and I feel a little relieved that maybe she and Sim can work things out on their own—without me having to teach her about transcendental sex. I say a hasty prayer. Nicky apparently feels the opposite and hisses under her breath something that sounds like "swine!"

When we're finished we go back to the Fire House to eat and Nicky fixes us a breakfast beyond belief: French toast drowning in berries, cinnamon and honey, eggs scrambled with tomatoes and peppers. She even finds enough champagne left from last night's dinner to make mimosas.

"Hungry?" I tease her, and she laughs.

"I have an incredible appetite, Dr. Jain," she replies with a wicked grin. "I'm ravenous."

In less than 15 minutes, there's not a morsel remaining on the table. I'm sorry Nat missed breakfast but I'm not sorry she misses what comes next.

Dave leans over and stares fondly at the partially completed lily pond puzzle. He starts to take it apart and put it back in the box. Nicky objects that it's not done yet and they need to wait for Prince to finish it.

"No, Nicky," Dave says firmly. "It's mine. I'm going to take it next door and play with my nurse. She's very disturbed. You should come with me."

"You're going to play with Brandy? She's a bitch, Dave. She hurt S&M. I don't want you to go."

"That's not nice, Nicky," he snarls. "That's not a nice way to talk about her. She could be your mother-in-law if you let her."

"That will be a cold day in hell, honey!" she hisses. "If she's your mother, then you're fucking around with your father!"

"I'm not fucking him, Nicky, you are. I'm just sharing."

They've only been married two months and I have a sinking feeling I'm seeing marriages unravel all around me as their tone escalates.

"If you're going to play with that snake then I'm going to go and play with your father. S&M loves me."

"He won't play with you like that, Nicky. He loves me much more than he loves you. He won't do it without me. Maybe he'll let you hit him though if you beg nicely."

He picks the puzzle box up and gives her a very mean little boyish smile. He's winning the fight.

"You should sit down and behave, Nicky," he sneers. "Be a good girl and don't make me lock you up."

He goes out the back door with his toy and she snorts like an angry stallion and moans, "Ooooh!" She doesn't seem to have strong enough words to express her anger.

I put a hand on her shoulder but I don't say anything. She's as tough as nails and much too hard to cry. When she regains her composure, she starts to swear quietly.

"The little bastard! I've done everything he asked."

"Nicky," I try to soothe her, "he's only going to entertain her with the puzzle. She's taken such good care of him and she's miserable right now. He's being very kind. What looks like cruelty to you is only your perception. He loves you more than anything.

"Stay here and we'll play dice. For money or for clothes, your choice."

Her eyes light up and a smile creeps into the corner of her mouth. "For clothes? Doctor Jain? You?"

"I'm not shy, Nicky," I say. "I know the difference between sex and love and lust. It's only a game, sweetheart. You can't lose."

Just then Nat walks in the kitchen door looking very distraught. "What's going on with you two?" she asks.

"Strip dice," I tell her. "Are you in or out?"

"Strip dice?" she thinks for a nanosecond. "Oh, baby I'm all the way in. I'm in up to my eyeballs."

†

DJ

Nim is my teacher and he's always right. Now I know exactly what he meant when he said women can be so demanding if you let them in. Nicky is a very good girl and a beautiful woman, but the more she gets, the hungrier she becomes.

Nim said I should know the difference between love and lust. I do know, but I can't understand how love without lust would be any smarter than lust without love. They fit together very nicely like the puzzle. I have to think hard about this one.

Brandy is upstairs in the nurses' room reading a little book when I get there. She opens the door and gives me a sweet kiss and then I understand it. Intimacy without sex. Love without lust. I love her very, very much but I don't want her. I love Nim much, much more and I want him to have her.

"I thought you might like to play, Brandy," I say showing her the puzzle. "It's a very good one. We almost had it solved yesterday but Prince had to go shopping and it takes a very long time. I can play with you for a little while and I can leave it here with you if you want to keep going."

I look around the room and it's only got a little desk and a chair and a bed, so I sit down in the middle of the floor and spread the pieces out. She sits down cross-legged across from me and we start sorting the pieces, looking for corners and flat edges, for bright colors and smooth patterns and any kind of clues.

It's a very wicked puzzle but she's the one who picked it out for me and now she gets to see just how hard it's going to be. The one I have has weeping willows hanging over the lily pond and it's hard to tell which of the green pieces are part of the tree and which are reflections in the water.

While we work I ask her what went wrong with Nim and she starts to cry. I don't even try to stop her. Crying works very nicely. But it's hard for her to talk and cry at the same time, so she finally sniffs it back.

"I did something very bad, Kama Dave," she sniffs. "I gave him your anti-psychotics and raped him. I lost control, baby."

"Brandy, that's very terrible. He might like the rape part but he really hates drugs. And he likes consciousness very much. I guess you just have to be punished."

"I know. I know. As long as it takes. I'm happy to be punished as long as he doesn't send me away."

"You need to learn about better sex, Brandy. The first thing Nat taught me about sex," I explain, "is control. She said if it's all physical, it's just animal sex. You should fuck his soul, not his body."

She stops trying to find a home for her puzzle piece and stares at me curiously. "How?"

"Well, I'm not going to show you how to do it, but maybe I can explain it to you. You have to see past the frosting, past the body, and tune into the breath and the heartbeat. And then you have to feel all his chakras before you even move.

"Maybe you never even move at all. Maybe you just look into his eyes until you can see his soul. You've got to get very, very intimate, inside the physical layer."

"Do you mean the koshas?"

"Right. You only use the body to access the energy and the mind and then you dive down into the heart and soul for the cake. If you do that, you'll have control of yourself and he'll trust you."

"Oh," she says. "It sounds complicated. How do you even learn how to do that?"

"Start by no sex at all. Just looking. Breathing. Go slow. Wait until he begs you, Brandy. It's worth waiting for. Pay attention to the fire at the beginning and avoid the embers in the end. Once you've got trust you've got everything. Once you lose it you've got nothing."

She nods and puts her attention back on the puzzle.

"Go slow until you find where the pieces belong. As long as it takes, Brandy. Put the pieces of the puzzle in the right places."

She concentrates on the little bit of the frame we've managed to piece together and gets on her knees to reach for another piece. The door opens and we both look up to see Nim standing there. He looks a little surprised to see us playing on the floor.

"Hmmph," he grunts. "You're still on your knees?"

"Yes, Sir," she whispers.

"Should I leave, Nim?" I ask politely.

"No. I think I'd much rather have you stay," he says quietly and sits down on the floor next to me, picking up a green piece. "This is a tricky piece," he laughs. "This one is the reflection in the water. It actually goes upside down. Right here," he says, placing it.

Brandy sits back on her heels and watches him. He looks up and glances at her for a second and then goes back to the puzzle. But I see him looking again with quick and careful flashes. Every time she sees him look at her, she forgets to breathe and I start laughing.

"Breathe," I coax her.

"What?" Nim looks at me. "What's going on here, Dave?"

"I'm teaching her control, Nim. Sex lessons."

"Fuck, Kamadev, what? Sex lessons?"

"Well, not like that, Nim. I'm teaching her with the puzzle. One piece at a time. I don't have sex with *your* wife, Nim. Not unless you beg me."

His mouth drops and then he laughs and punches me in the arm. He looks at Brandy curiously.

"Just what has delirious Dave taught you about sex, Bran?"

She blushes but she looks him straight in the eye and says, "Start with no sex and wait as long as it takes. Don't fuck your body; wait until I can feel your soul. Maybe don't move at all, just look and breathe. Wait until you beg."

He stares at her without blinking and then his mouth twists in amusement. "Damn," he snorts. "Interesting."

He goes back to the puzzle, but he keeps looking up to check on her.

"What are you reading, Bran?" he finally asks, seeing the little book open on the bed.

"The Jewel," she says. "*The self-controlled man enjoys eternal bliss*," she quotes.

"Shankara?" he's stunned.

"Mack loaned it to me. I'm reading *you*, Sim. I'm reading your soul."

"Hmmm," he purrs and his eyes narrow like lasers focusing on their target.

I put my hand on his back behind his heart and he turns to look at me. "Good work, Kamadev," he smiles. "You may be able to keep your nurse after all."

"She'll study hard, Nim," I promise him. "She's a very good straight A student. Give her another test."

"Alright then," he sighs. "I might help her finish the puzzle, Kamadev. Uh—alone. If you help me any more we could *really* confuse her."

†

BRANDY

Kama Dave gets to his feet and leaves the nurses' room with a self-satisfied smile, well deserved for the little Cupid that he is. Sim goes back to the task at hand, gently picking out the pieces he prefers, concentrating on the weeping willow reflections in the pond.

In between placing the pieces, he looks up and gives me a searing look deep into my soul, each time a little longer, a little warmer. The ice in his eyes is gradually melting but instead of feeling passion and lust rise in me, I feel fear, the dread of being parted from him.

"What else did he teach you, Bran?" he asks looking at the floor again.

I think carefully and say, "He said to pay attention to the fire at the beginning in order to avoid the embers at the end. I'm not sure exactly what that means."

"Well, think about it. What do you think it means?"

"A fire starts out blazing and warm and ends up cold and dead with very little heat. It's used up its fuel. Maybe it means to keep stoking the fire so it doesn't burn out."

"It's a Tantric verse, Brandy. What it means is that if you tend the fire instead of trying to burn up all the fuel you can maintain the warmth and keep it going. The fire is your prana, your life energy. The fuel is your sexual desire.

"If your goal is to consummate the act of sex, to finish it off and release the tensions of desire, you kill the energy of the fire.

"But if you stay in the present and practice intimate awareness without going anywhere, the fire can burn indefinitely, the heat builds instead of dissipates.

"The point is, do you want to tend the fire or do you just want to burn up all the wood?"

He looks up again and watches me carefully.

"I want the fire to burn, Sim, not the wood," I answer. "I want it to burn for a long time, forever."

"Good," he smiles. "I wrote that letter because I saw something very disturbing in you this morning, desperate hunger and lust. Now I'm seeing something else in your eyes. Curiosity.

Maybe even a little wonder. Come over here," he beckons.

He's sitting cross-legged on the floor in his leather pants and as I rise, he motions for me to sit on his lap.

"With all my clothes?" I ask.

"Absolutely with all your clothes," he laughs. "You are a little nuclear warhead, Brandy. I need some protection from your radioactivity."

I sit down carefully on his lap wrapping my legs around his waist and put my hands on his beautiful shoulders. He doesn't kiss me but he puts his hands on my back, above and below my heart and gazes into my eyes.

"Just like this, beautiful girl," he whispers. "As long as it takes. Or until my legs fall asleep," he laughs.

I gaze into his right eye and then the left and I feel the heat of his body in my hands and on my back. An hour ago he was lost to me forever and now I hold him like the irreplaceable treasure that he is.

We just sit together, not moving, just breathing and I drink him in. Slowly and steadily his eyes deepen into reflecting pools and seem to change from gunmetal blue to green and silver. I can see the images of weeping willows dripping onto still water and see white water lilies floating on the surface of his irises.

I feel his heart beating in his fingertips and feel his breath flowing from his nose onto my neck. I'm afraid to move even the least bit lest I disturb the surface of the pond. I breathe in time to him and watch his face dissolve in quiet passion, his eyes glazed with ecstasy and bliss.

Soft waves of pleasure begin to rise up my spinal cord through my heart. I can feel his sex inside me pulsing through my fingers and toes, rising to my throat, throbbing in my head. My entire existence is ignited and my body quietly disappears into a river of fire. My mind simply wanders away.

I hear the door open and some words and it closes but it matters not a bit anymore. I am entirely inside of him, consumed by him. I am the pulse that beats his heart and the air that breathes him.

†

## MACK

It's late in the afternoon and Sunny has gone down the mountain to shop, so I decide to stretch my legs and walk over to the pool house to check on my little brother. He's really been troubling me since he disappeared a few days ago; he seems more unstable than ever. There's no answer but the door is open so I go out back and check the yoga deck.

Two mats are laid out, one in teaching position, and I smile. If he's been teaching, he hasn't dropped the connection.

There's no one by the pool or in the gym, so I head next door to the Fire House. I can hear a lot of laughter before I even open the door and it sounds nice.

The kitchen is a bit of a mess with empty wine bottles, open cracker boxes and hunks of cheese. It sounds like there's a party going on in the boardroom.

Jain, Nat, Kama Dave and Nicky are all gathered around the big table drinking wine and playing dice. Apparently, by the state of their lack of attire, it's strip dice.

Dave's wearing nothing but a braided leather belt, Nat has a prayer shawl and panties and Dr. Jain is in his boxers. Nicky is fully dressed with a nice little collection of clothing draped over the back of her chair including leather pants, a couple kimonos, pretty plum colored yoga pants, a plum lace camisole and some black sweat pants.

When I come in Nicky turns around and takes a look at my clothes and sucks on her lower lip, deciding whether she needs a pair of old khaki hospital scrubs. I read her mind.

"No, Nicky," I laugh. "I'm just looking for Steven. Do I need to put out another APB for him?"

"Isn't he at his house?" she sulks.

"Nah," Dave says, "he's upstairs, Doc, at your house playing with the puzzle. He's fine."

Nicky's eyes narrow but not before I see the blazing green goddess of jealousy burning inside them.

"Thanks, guys," I laugh. "It's a little too hot in here for me. See you later."

It's quiet at my house when I return and I listen at the door of the upstairs room before I knock. If Steven and Brandy are working things out, I don't want to interrupt. But if he's flown off the handle again and taken off I need to know sooner rather than later.

I don't hear anything. I knock and no one answers. I try the door and its unlocked so I open it quietly. The air tastes of jasmine and sandalwood. It's not really a scent; it's a subtle flavor of flowers, a taste permeating the space. The room is deathly quiet.

In the middle of the floor Steven is sitting with Brandy on his lap fully dressed. Neither of them is moving, possibly not even breathing they are so still. Her back is to me but I can see his face is vacant, his eyes dilated into black pools ringed with blue edges staring at her in a trance of rapture.

My first thought is 'what drugs are they on now?' Then I notice a high frequency in the room all the way from the doorway and a light energy that pours into my navel center. I feel like I'm being covered with tender light kisses from all sides.

It's the most intimate and erotic sight I've ever seen but there is nothing moving, nothing doing, nowhere going. They're not even present in the room.

I apologize quickly although nobody seems to be there and take a deep breath in before I close the door. I can taste Kama, the essence of love. My legs are shaky from the impact of the vision, so I go down the stairs carefully and take refuge in my office.

The ribald gambling, drinking and nudity at Jain's house was charged with lewdness, levity and rivalry but there was nothing even subliminally sexual. What I just witnessed upstairs has taken my breath away with its pure ethereal eroticism.

I feel my stomach growl and my heart pounds. A new form of hunger in me begs for nourishment.

†

NICK

The party is just getting started. Dr. Jain and Nat are experiencing a little bit of beginners luck as we trade a few articles of clothing back and forth. The ladies definitely have the upper hand over Dr. Jain as we have jewelry to put into the betting pool before we actually lose any of our clothes.

The newlyweds are still floating in the clouds from the night before and blissfully regaling the details of the elaborate feast served by the little Prince. They have my mouth watering so bad, I dig around in the kitchen fridge and cupboards and find cheese, crackers, nuts and a nice stash of wine.

Dr. Jain is a beautiful man and even though he's not available I get immense pleasure just being in his company. I also like Nat quite a bit. Her energy is very similar to S&M's. As his assistant therapist, she's intimate with him in the same kind of relationship I used to have: BS, Before Sex.

I'm enjoying their company so much that I forget my feud with Kama Dave. That is, until he comes back into the house with a smug little smile on his innocent face, looking like he controls the Universe and all of its minions. He's becoming more arrogant than S&M in that department.

He's got nothing on but his leathers and a crystal pendant and I'm betting I can take everything he's got in three rolls of the dice. I feel the heat of anger rising and he's arousing a singularly different appetite in me with his domineering attitude. I'm going to take him down.

"Oooh, dice," he purrs. "I love games."

I love games too baby, I think to myself. Some more than others. I'm going to make up some new rules and teach them to him very clearly and methodically, just like I used to play with S&M. Game On.

Shiva Dice is one of S&M's favorite past-times and I've played it with him for years. I know it inside out and, although it's a game of chance, if another player is not paying attention, it's pretty easy to play crooked.

The rules are a little twisted so a player might not realize he has the winning toss. If it slides by,

I'm not going to correct anyone. Dave knows the rules though and once he sits down with us, I just have to cross my fingers and play fair.

By the time Dr. Mack comes in looking for S&M, I'm well ahead of everyone. Too bad he doesn't want to play. I'd like to dress Kama Dave up in those old hospital scrubs and play doctor with him. Ah, well.

I ply Dave with a little wine and then win his last piece, the leather belt.

"Game over, baby," I tease. "You haven't got anything left to bargain with but your favors and not everyone here at the table is going to be willing to place a value on that."

Nat blushes furiously and Dr. Jain laughs a little nervously.

"Oooh noooo," Dave moans. "It can't be over that fast. I haven't got them here, but I'll wager my favorite raggedy jeans if you let me play some more."

Nat and Dr. Jain still have a bit of game left so I assent, but when Dave loses on the next roll he's got nothing left to his name but some cash and a lot of love potions and oils. He can't even come to the dinner table now unless he wears a bath towel.

"You've got to give me my leather pants back, Nicky," he begs. "You know I got them to entertain you. I have plans."

Nat and Dr. Jain are roaring with laughter, not at his nakedness but at his helpless dependence, reduced to begging.

"Nicky please," he pleads again.

I throw him Dr. Jain's black gym sweats instead. "Cover yourself up, baby," I sneer. "I own you now."

"No, Nicky, no! Nim bought the leathers for me so I could entertain you. Please! You don't know what you're missing."

"Oh, you're entertaining me very much right now, baby Dave. I'm not missing anything."

I pretend to ignore him and thank Nat for the beautiful plum lace trimmed yoga outfit. My wardrobe is next to nothing and it's a very nice and expensive looking addition.

"May I try it on, Nat?" I ask and she shrugs.

"Go on, Nicky. It's yours now. We had fun. Who knows? I may win it back again someday."

I slip the plum suit on under my dress in a beach change without even leaving the room. It feels nice and tight and shows off my bodybuilder parts: calves, chest, shoulders and arms. Dr. Jain whistles in approval. Dave gives me a pitiful crooked frown.

"I guess the game is over," Nat laughs. "For now."

"It's just starting," I laugh. "But the kimonos belong to the house so I'm not going to take them." I give them back to Nat and Jain and they push away from the table and go back to their room to put some more clothes on. Or not.

I feel a wave of power and hunger roll through me as I look down at Dave sulking in his used sweat pants, a couple sizes too big to fit. I pick up my new fringe leather belt and wrap one end of it around my knuckles.

"I may be inclined to give this belt back to you though, baby Dave," I growl snapping the belt lightly against the boardroom tabletop. "I'd really like to give it to you a lot. Maybe six or seven times. Then we can negotiate about the pants."

†

## S&M

It's nearly dark by the time I bring my awareness back to the room. I notice her eyes are as wide as saucers, the pupils deep black pools, and the dark brown irises have turned shimmering gold, more the color of butter than chocolate. Her breath is indiscernible.

I could stay with her like this for an eternity but my legs are twitching with pins and needles as they come back from sleep. I give her a little squeeze and whisper.

"Sweet girl, it's time to get off me."

Her eyes drift and then focus on me and I see myself reflected in those golden pools.

"Oh, Sim!" she gasps. "Was that—?"

"Just the beginning," I growl. "You passed the entrance exam."

I help her up and then massage my legs to get the blood back into them. When she sees what I'm doing she drops back down to her knees and helps me, gently squeezing my thighs and calves and kneading my feet.

It's not sexual but it's so compassionate that I groan and lie back on the floor, trusting her to touch me. She keeps it therapeutic, massaging like a nurse, staying away from the erogenous zones, concentrating on my feet, ankles and calves.

"Is it okay, Sim?" she asks. "I want to learn what you like."

"It's beautiful, gorgeous," I sigh. "Keep it up."

"Did that satisfy you?" she asks after a long pause. "Do you really prefer not having straight sex? Because I will do anything or nothing if that's what pleases you."

"Very satisfying, Bran," I murmur. "But there's much more to it. It's complicated. If you want to do this with me, you have to be patient. You have to be willing to wait as long as it takes, maybe forever. There's no goal, baby. It's just a beautiful trip that ends up right back where we started."

I sit up again and hold both of her hands.

"Brandy, you don't know me. You don't know who I am. You were a brazen girl to marry a stranger. What were you thinking?"

"I was thinking you were the most delicious man I'd ever seen. An arrogant, conceited, rich bastard with a bad reputation who would be worth any amount of trouble."

It's pretty apt and I'm deeply amused at that.

"You knew my reputation?" I smirk.

"I had heard about you. Hundreds of girls, Sir. None of them treated very nicely or kindly but most likely none of them left with any regrets for having had, uh—made your acquaintance.

"When I met Nicky, when you were in the hospital, she told me you were celibate, that you'd given up sex but were still very kinky. I thought the challenge was even more interesting."

"That woman ought to watch her mouth," I groan. "I've been trying to clean up my act for years and I don't need that kind of gossip, even if it's true. There's nothing worse than celibacy to generate perversity. I won't even begin to mention how freaky Nicky can get."

I let go of her hands and pout, remembering how close I was to Nick, how I submitted to her games and let her win just to keep the dice rolling and the world turning. And now—man, I'll bet she'll be pretty pissed at me if I turn my back on her now, if I quit playing in her threesome.

Aw, the times I turned my back on her before so she could lay into me with a lash and I just laughed because I felt no pain. How powerful she felt having the man of her dreams on his knees, the illusion of control. How easy it was for me to play because I gave up nothing; it only strengthened my own resolve and self-control.

"May I, Sir?" Brandy asks politely and I see her face is inches from mine now. I sniff and nod and she kisses me on my forehead then lightly on my lips. I sigh was satisfaction and look around.

"Ah, the nurses' room," I laugh. "Shitty little bed you have isn't it? I guess I've inconvenienced you with this punishment."

"That's the least of it, Sim. I'd sleep on rocks if you'd forgive me," she says, searching my face for a clue. "Sunny and I used to fight over who got the bed. The loser had to sleep on a cot. The lumpy bed is a very mild punishment."

I laugh and get up to my feet and look down on her. I start untying the belt in a subtle strip tease. I'm going to give her the midterm exam.

"Would this bother you too much, nurse? Can you keep your head?"

"Oh, god, Sim," she pants. "Yes. I can. I mean no it won't. Oh, shit."

"Come on, honey," I tease her. "I'm just getting started with this. I've got forever. Do you want to be patient with me or should I go home?"

She drops her eyes and says, "Patience." Then she looks back up and watches me playing with her, stripping purposely and chastely without a hint of wicked suggestion. I want to make this easy so she doesn't spontaneously combust.

I climb under the covers of the shitty little nurses' bed and close my eyes. I could sleep so easily. If I did yoga nidra right now I'd drop off the edge of the earth within three minutes.

I feel her swim into my arms, soft and warm. I wrap myself around her with my mouth on her neck and drop back into those deep golden pools where she lies floating inside the echo of my snores and I'm gone.

†

DJ

"Nicky, no," I tell her firmly once we're up in our room. Maybe Nim will buy me some more clothes. I feel foolish for gambling but I can't let her have the upper hand. She's my prisoner and I don't want to negotiate control with her.

"Baby Dave," she purrs, "you know I would never hurt you. You've done this before. You liked it."

She's dangling my handcuffs in front of me, and trying to make a deal. I don't like it. It's one thing to play and an entirely different scene to be forced. It scares me.

"Why do you have the handcuffs if you don't want to play with them, baby?" she continues.

"It's for a different game, Nicky. A surprise. I might show you if you give me my clothes back."

I realize I can't even do a strip tease for her now because I haven't got anything to take off except for Dr. Jain's lousy old gym pants. They could just as easily fall off me than work for a strip.

But she doesn't quit. She comes up close to me, close enough that I can feel her heat, and turns her green cat eyes on me.

"I want to do this, Kamadev," she hisses. "I miss it. S&M used to play with me all the time. I want you on your knees, baby."

"I don't like that game, Nicky," I whine. "I don't like being locked up and abused. It's not fun for me. Can't we play something else?"

She snorts and puts her hand down on me and squeezes my cock so hard it hurts.

"You little bastard," she swears. "You may look like him but you're just a baby. Oh! Look at you! Are you really going to start crying now? I can't believe it, you little crybaby!"

I sniff. Maybe I *will* start crying. Crying works very nicely especially with psychos. Then I remember the handcuffs are mine.

"I'll trade you the handcuffs, Nicky," I sniff.

"Well now, what would I do with the damn handcuffs if you refuse to play?"

"You can wear them. I'd be happy to play with the handcuffs on you. I might like that."

She swears again.

"Okay. No handcuffs then. But will you please play? Just hold the chair like you did before."

"No," I say. "I don't feel like being hit today. You're too hungry right now, Nicky. You might kill me."

"Don't tempt me, honey," she hisses.

She throws herself into the chair in despair and pouts. She looks like she needs to cry but I don't think she knows how. Her eyes are as dark as the forest and I think I've hurt her but I don't know why. I love her.

She looks like a goddess in the purple lace stretchy suit. I want her to kiss me and be happy but she's horribly frustrated with me. But I'm not Nim. I don't want to be his substitute; I don't want to play the same old games he played with her. Whips and chains are so old fashioned, so coarse, like junk food sex.

I want to seduce her with nourishment and love. Instead of putting sugar in the medicine, I want to just give her the sugar, to give her so much pleasure that she loses her desire to cause me pain.

She looks so horribly lost and sad right now as if she doesn't know what to do with her self. I think she's become too hungry to be satisfied with even the most perfect apple. She's thinking of all the junk she can fill herself up with just to be full of herself.

What can the God of Love do to fill her up with love arrows again I wonder? Think, Kamadev! I furrow my forehead in deep sympathy and close my eyes. I hear Nim teaching me, 'You are the present. It's going to make her scream!' I see the image of Shiva Nataraj dancing and trampling the little body of the ignorant dwarf, the ego. That's it, I think. I have to crush her with the dance.

"Nicky," I offer. "I don't need these gym pants. You can have them back."

She glares at me and frowns.

I take the handcuffs from her and snap them on my wrist like Nim does, both bracelets doubled up on one side. And then I just pretend I have all my assets and accessories. It's all the illusion of Maya anyway.

I pretend I have a blessing scarf around my shoulders and I slide it very sexy back and forth across my back until I get her attention. And then I swing nothing around and around over my head and toss it at her. She looks very confused.

I pretend I'm taking my kimono off, opening one side and touching my chest, then covering it up again. Opening the other side, admiring my chest and touching myself like I'm made out of solid gold. I lock eyes with her and lick my lips and pretend to slide the imaginary silk off my shoulders.

I see her green eyes dilating now as she starts to understand my make believe strip tease. Her sweet mouth twists into a smile and she shows a few teeth as she realizes the game; her face begins to sparkle. Sex starts in the heart and mind. The imagination is the greatest aphrodisiac.

I pull the pretend belt out of my imaginary leather pants and wrap the end around my knuckles and whack my open palm gently and then lash the bed hard with the pretend fringed end, biting down on my lip. I make a face at her like I'd love to bite her head off and have fun doing it.

I nearly give the whole act away without having the tools I need, without the music or the clothes. All I have is the sheer will to entertain her with all my heart.

When I finally get down to the last part, the ugly old sweatpants, I give her a real tease, turning my back on her and flashing a bit of my ass, covering it up, turning back to her and pulling the sweats low enough to show a little pubic hair but nothing more.

She's laughing and clapping now and I'm bumping my hips to an imaginary drumbeat. I turn my back again and show her the full moon, cover my ass and then I turn around, tapping my foot impatiently while I count to ten before I drop everything. Nim taught me well.

I can see all her teeth now and hear her breathing hard and heavy. I step out of the sweat pants on the floor and put my hand around my erection, admiring it and giving myself a couple slow respectful celebratory strokes.

"I'm not a baby," I snarl at her.

Now the dance has turned the game around and she's starting to disintegrate. She gets down on the floor and covers my bare feet with kisses. I pull her hair so she has to stand on her knees face to face with my manhood.

She looks up at me with her dark green eyes blazing with lust and she groans, "No, you're not a baby."

Then she puts me in her mouth and sucks softly. She's the baby. While she's busy with that, I unlock the handcuffs and snap them on her wrists and then pull her up to her feet.

I realize it's impossible now to take her lace camisole off because she's cuffed, so I pull the straps down around her arms and pull the rest of it down around her waist to free her breasts.

She's all tangled up now in lace and handcuffs and it's very complicated looking. I snort and giggle at the same time because I like it very much. I push her down on the bed and look at the mess I've made.

She's a very nice looking puzzle and it will be a real pleasure to solve it. She can't even put her arms around me unless I unlock her and I don't want to. She looks dangerous, like a wild animal, but she's not mad at me anymore. She's ravenous, restrained and ready.

I think she would frighten me like this if she weren't so tangled up, but right now she is my willing toy, my beautiful baby doll.

"These new stretchy pants are very sexy on you, Nicky," I growl as I strip them off slowly and carefully. "Very beautiful, but they're in my way."

I turn her on her side and lie face to face so her bound hands can touch me and play with me. I kiss her hard stroking her beautiful ass. I like this new game very much. I'll bet she's never played like this before. How would she even think of doing it like this? How could she even know the rules? I'm making them up!

I make her go slow and easy with her hands so I can tease her for a long time, biting her and pulling her hair gently. I growl at her and laugh and she starts whimpering with desire.

"Now don't cry, darling baby girl," I scold her. "I'm going to take very good care of you. I have something special just for you today, something you never tried before. Kama Dave's special psycho sex."

Then I turn her over with her back to me and take her that way so my hands are free to roam all over the front of her. I can tell by all her incoherent moaning and screaming that her mind is being destroyed.

I have to put one hand over her mouth to keep the noise down. Then I stop moving altogether to get her full attention.

"Nicky?" I command her, "You'll stop calling me Baby Dave. Do you understand?"

"Yes, Sir," she says. "Please don't stop yet, honey."

I give her some more very nice slow strokes and say, "Honey is fine or Sugar. Kama Dave or Sri Dave is fine, but no more Baby Dave. Understood?"

"Yes, Sri Psycho Dave Sugar," she complies. "No more Baby. Whatever pleases you, honey," she moans and groans.

I wonder what else I can make her do now. I have a few ideas but the way it's going right now is really much too sweet and psychotic, so I just keep it up. I keep it up until long after the sun has gone down. I keep it up until I smell dinner.

†

## NAT

Prince shows up at sunset with a big box of produce and some beautiful crab, sour dough bread and more wine. How he managed to buy the alcohol at the young age of 18 is beyond me but I suspect it has to do with his expense account. Then again I wonder, how did he get his hands on ounces on heroin when he was twelve years old? I'm not going to push it.

He steams the crab and makes an awesome lemon aioli dip and salad, but the heavenly scent doesn't really rise in the house until he puts the sour dough under the broiler with garlic butter spiced with paprika, cumin and turmeric.

As if on cue, Nicky descends the staircase looking like a ravishing playmate, dressed in my former plum lace yoga outfit. I have to admit she makes the clothes even more beautiful with her voluptuous curves. Both Prince and Rick stop to drink in the vision.

On her heals, his royal haughtiness Kamadev is dressed to the nines in black leather pants, braided belt, crystal pendant, saffron silk kimono, white prayer scarf, fingerless gloves, and damn if he doesn't have the little silver handcuff necklace back around his neck again. And he's barefoot of course.

Apparently his clothing negotiations have succeeded with whatever favors he offered in trade. If only Sim could see him now I think, he'd be proud of his prize student, but Sim never shows for dinner.

†

## BRANDY

Expectation is the root of all heartache according to Shakespeare, but I have no expectations at all so I don't mind it when Sim passes out in my arms and snores. I would die twice just to have him sleeping in my arms again. I will wait as long as it takes for the rest.

He's such a confusing belligerent compassionate being. I fall into deep sleep with him and dream I'm wandering in his veins and beating his heart and kissing his mind. And then I dream he is fully inside me, softly stroking every inch of me.

I dream sex better than I any sex I've ever known. I dream orgasms one after the other over and over until I wake myself up groaning and realize I'm really having them. He's sleeping inside me, fucking me in his dreams.

I don't remember how this got started but I'm not composing a letter of complaint. I feel his orgasms pouring through me. He's coming. I'm coming. No one is driving. The Universe is burning. We're coming over and over like a broken record. I fall into him and sink back into dream sex.

At the far side of a lake there are deep marshes with graceful grasses and bright mango lilies floating downstream, fallen, dead, spent. I'm floating in his arms at his mercy. He breathes and the world turns. He puts his foot down in the dance, crushing the insolence, the egos, the ignorance, the ashes.

Ah, he puts his foot down and comes even harder.

†

## SEAN

I'm on the Board of Directors at Sunrise, head of the screening committee, so I have to think pretty hard about doing this. I know their focus is on wellness care and so far I've brought them a junkie and a derelict drunk, both of them personal friends.

The new guy is going to turn their reality on its head if I take him up there. I feel the double-edged sword of guardianship and responsibility but I haven't really got a choice in the matter.

I call Mack first to run it by him.

"Shit, Sean!" he swears. "I think I'd rather have a dozen more junkies than get into this. Steven is off the rails with his personal issues."

"Okay," I acquiesce, "it could ruin your whole scene up there. If you don't want to be bothered, I can get him into something more conventional."

I wait and listen. Silence is the most powerful persuasion I know. I don't want to press it but if Mack doesn't take this guy I know he's lost.

"Are you sure, Sean?" he asks. If there was ever a more compassionate man than Dr. Mack, I've yet to meet him. I can hear him caving in.

"Oh, brother, no doubt about it," I say. "You can see for yourself tomorrow if you're willing to meet him. I just don't want to bring him up there unless you know what you're getting into."

He's silent for a minute and then he laughs with resignment. "Bring it on, Sean. It's why we're here."

†

## MAC

It's quiet for a change on the top of the mountain, as if the page is being turned on a finished chapter. I think about my little brother and one of the clearest images that comes to mind is Steven sitting on the office couch with his dirty feet up on the table, his soles freshly covered with the forest floor peat and pine, brooding over his youthful excesses and indiscretions.

Oh, man. Things are about to get wild up here. I need to give him a fair warning about what's coming up, but tomorrow morning is soon enough. What he's up to in the nurses' room upstairs is far more important for his health and wellbeing. And I need him well and stable.

I put my feet up on the table like he did. My poor feet have loafers on them and I kick them off in sympathetic contempt. Sunny comes into the office to check on me and raises an eyebrow at my bare feet on the table.

"Would you like to join me for dinner at the Fire House?" I invite her. "It's been a long time since we've been over there and Jain has been raving about the little chef's cuisine. Trust me honey, we need to relax while we still can."

When we walk in through the kitchen, Prince beams with pride. He's already got the salad and main course on the table and he's fussing with some mango crème brulee coming out of the oven.

Nat and Jain are radiant. It's our third wedding in three months and I resolve to join them soon. I just want to wait a little while until the surface chop calms down up here.

Kama Dave and Nicky are seated at the table feeding each other bits of crab and sough dough with total absorption and adoration. God, I've seen that before. I've seen it with Steven and Brandy and then I've seen it dissipate in the ashes of passion. I've been there with my dead wife. It hurts to watch it.

I wince and look at Sunny. We barely know each other. It's only been three months. If I want to get there from here, back to the core of the universe, back to love, I have to work on it harder. I need to take the time to know her better.

Dave is overjoyed to see me. He jumps up and squeezes the air out of me with a bear hug. Then he teases me about living in sin with Sunny and starts joking about the times I shot up morphine with him.

"Doc! Mack. You were the Man! I loved it. I would have never quit except Nim said I couldn't play with him in the gym and the pool and the yoga deck. It was a hard call, Doctor Feelgood. A very hard call," he laughs.

"Aw, yeah. I almost forgot about prison! But God bless me when my rehab is up in four months," he continues. "It's going to be another very hard call, man!"

I hope to hell he's joking. I hope very hard because there's only the thinnest veil separating me from morphine now and the last thing I need is a shooting gallery buddy. Especially one who looks just like my brother.

I blush in front of God and Jain. I blush in front of Sunny, Nat and Nicky. And then I look hopelessly up at Prince, the innocent little retired heroin dealer, who is serving me a sweet crème brulee. I skip the main course and go straight for the dessert.

There's only the thinnest veil separating me from bliss or despair, the veil of humanity. I nod and respond politely to the conversations around me and take a few bites of crab, a few sips of wine, but more than anything I drink the humanity around the boardroom table.

Kama Dave looks so much like my brother. I remember Steven asking me if I might have had a child when I was 15, if maybe Dave could be his nephew. It's impossible. But I've been wondering if Dad had one on the side. Dad was pretty wild and died very young. Steven was 13. I was 21. Dave would've been 6. My head spins.

I look at Nicky, but I have to turn away. She looks like a centerfold and she's completely engrossed doting on Dave. I blow all my air out and gaze at Sunny for grounding, but she's also enraptured in the veil of Maya.

Nat is radiating bliss and when I look to my dear old friend and colleague Jain he just shakes his head from side to side with experiential joy.

"Mack, oh Mack," he breathes. "Yes, yes, yes! You absolutely have to dine with us more often, man!"

"I will, Jain," I promise. I spend far too much time alone.

There is a deep grief in me, and a deep relief, a tumultuous mix. Nothing can be changed, nothing can be 'fixed'. Everything that remains is a momentary gift, a blessing, and there is no hope that anything will last.

I remember the ancient Sufi story of the king who asked his wise men to find a truth which would be appropriate in all times and situations. They presented him with a ring that made happy men sad and sad men happy, simply engraved with the words 'And this, too, shall pass away.'

Abraham Lincoln quoted that story in one of his speeches with the comment, 'How chastening in the hour of pride! How consoling in the depths of affliction!'

My mind drifts off and suddenly it's filled with a clear vision that sends chills through me. Even if it isn't true, the horror of it perforates my heart.

When our parents died, they were quite wealthy. In addition to an immense insurance policy, which paid double indemnity for accidental death, I inherited the mountain top property. I spent a good chunk of money on med school and invested Steven's share.

When he turned 18, I co-signed for his beach house. His property value alone has increased nearly four times in the last ten years. Even before Steven started teaching yoga he was obscenely wealthy for a guy his age.

But Dave—if he is our half-brother, abandoned by Dad and his lover—Dave was left penniless.

I stare at Dave again and he's grinning back at me with his arm around his beautiful playmate, stroking her neck with his fingertips. He's a pretty sick boy and he would be in prison or a mental ward right now if Steven hadn't found him and taken him under his wing.

I try to soothe my horror—all's well that ends well, as the saying goes—but I know in my soul nothing ever ends. One man's indiscretion has caused so much pain and suffering for this kid if he's Dad's child.

Steven said he might have had 100 bastards before he turned 20. I multiply Dave's damage by a hundred and the magnitude of it hits me like a sucker punch. I begin to realize the enormity of the karmic guilt Steven's been trying to sort out.

I wonder how many kids Dad had? How many half-brothers and sisters do I have out there in the world? How many nieces and nephews—not even counting Steven's hundred? I stop breathing.

"Mack, honey?" Sunny whispers. "Are you ill? You're not eating."

I turn and stare at her. Could she be my sister, I wonder? No way. With red hair and freckles, not a chance. I breathe a little sigh of relief and resolve to help clean up Dad's mess and Steven's mess.

"No, I'm fine," I say. "The dessert filled me up. I'm just very, very thirsty." I smile and hold my empty glass out to Jain.

"Board meeting here at noon tomorrow," I remind him. "Sean is bringing a new guy up to meet the screening committee. It would be a good idea if everyone clears out of the house but the Board of Directors."

"Swimming!" Dave suggests with a sparkle and I can envision him lounging at the pool with Prince and all the beautiful ladies. His pure joy is contagious. I wish I had his simple presence and contentment. Maybe he wasn't dealt such a bad hand after all.

†

## S&M

At 6am we wake in synchronicity, my eyes on hers, my sex in hers, my heart and soul buried inside hers. So far, so good, I think. Maybe we can figure this out after all. I get up and go downstairs to fetch tea and fruit for us and Mack catches me in the kitchen.

"We need to talk brother," he says. "Board meeting at noon. Sean's coming up, but we need to talk before then."

"Cool, cool," I say. "Give me a little more time."

"You got it worked out?" he wonders. "I might need to get the nurses' room back. A new guy is coming up."

"Nothing like this gets worked out overnight, brother," I laugh. "It's a work in progress. I'll be down to see you at 10, okay?"

He looks pretty worried but my number one agenda item at the moment is this sweet girl who is trying so hard to be my wife. I serve her a little breakfast in bed and ask her to read the Shankara text to me. It's been a long time since I've heard the words and I relish her careful narrative. She enuniciates the Sanskrit cautiously.

*Brahma satyam jagat mithyā, jīvo brahmaiva nāparah*
'Creation is truth. Space and time are the illusion of separation between the self and the creator.'

I might have more fun playing dice and reading Sanskrit with her than this bedroom mayhem I've been trying to sort out. But from what I see in her eyes now, she'll play whatever I like. I'm beginning to hope and dream her again.

At ten, I rap on Mac's door and I feel pretty nice, ethereal and polished. He's got his bare feet up on the table and I laugh and do the same.

"Mack, you've been a damn good big brother," I laugh, "for better or for worse. I'm sorry I hit you with all my shit."

He pushes the bourbon decanter across the table to me. It's morning and I raise an eyebrow.

"You've been a damn good big brother, too," he laughs, "although you probably didn't realize it. We could do a DNA test on Dave but I don't think it's necessary."

"Fucking what?" I spit. "You said—"

"I said he couldn't be my kid, Steven."

He lets it sink in and then continues.

"You take after your father, Steven. He was a wild man. I was always very, very careful about sex because I saw how much he hurt our mother. She turned a blind eye on it because she loved him so much.

"You were much too young to notice. But he was very promiscuous. I'll bet my mountain house against your beach house that Dave is his."

He waits and watches for my reaction. My mind is racing and my heart is pacing it. I love it! I love DJ. But holy hell! I may have just slept with my brother and my brother's wife. I don't even want to know if that constitutes incest. I can't begin to tell Mack. I pour a lot of breakfast bourbon.

"Uhm," I say. "DNA?"

"Yeah, we can do sibling testing but without our parents it only gives a good probability of relationship. But I'd say just looking at the boy and his—um, behavior—tells the whole story. We can test him, but it's my educated opinion he's our half-brother.

"And judging by the way he's got that beautiful woman eating out of the palm of his hand, ten years older than he is, I'd say he takes after Dad too."

"Wow," I blow.

He watches and listens. That was always his strong point as a teacher, not preaching but absorbing.

"Sooooo," I wonder, "That's what this is all about?"

"Not even, Steven," he warns me. "I've saved the real shocker for last. Sean has a new stray who has been stalking the beach house. He can tell you the whole story, but in a nutshell, he's got a nine-year old kid who says his father lives there. Sean swears he's your spitting image.

"Unless you tell me otherwise, he'll be here at noon."

"Oh," I joke weakly, "there's only one?"

†

## SEAN

Jack is sitting in the back of the squad car playing with the handcuffs. His little fists are so small he can put them on and take them off without a key, the youngest little culprit I've escorted in the cage.

I hope to hell Sim is going to take him in because the alternative is not good. Crystal wants to keep him but that's legally impossible. The kid will end up in a foster home and it'll be the same old story as DJ and Prince: another runaway fucked up and living on the street.

"How high are we going, Officer?" he wonders. "I thought my father lived at the beach."

"All the way to the top, Jack. I live in your father's house now. He was hurt very bad and we brought him to the top of the mountain so he could get well."

"Is he hurt very much still?" he asks.

"He's much better," I say. "I think he'll be happy to see you."

"Does that mean I don't have to go to jail?"

"Not today, buddy. Not if you behave yourself."

"Yes, Sir. Officer."

He gets up on his knees on the seat to look out the back window at the ocean in the distance.

"I never been this high before," he marvels. "We're higher than the clouds."

I hit the siren once to announce myself when I pull in the driveway and get Jack out and take the handcuffs away from him.

"Aw," he moans.

"Nope. That's not a toy." It's not a toy unless you're over 21 and married I think, but I keep it to myself.

Sim opens the front door and just stands there, staring at us. Jack looks like he's going to run for the hills.

"Hey, Sim," I break the ice, "this is my buddy Jack. He's been snooping around your house for a couple days."

Sim nods his head with a dazed expression.

"Jack, this is Mr. Mack. I don't know what the hell you're supposed to call him but I'm sure he'll let you know."

Jack bites down on one of his fingers and doesn't move. Then Sim breaks out laughing.

"Jack Mack! That's too good. He sounds like a bruiser. Are you going to shake my hand or punch me, Jack?"

Jack takes his hand out of his mouth, walks up to the porch cautiously and sticks it out for a handshake.

"Cool," Sim laughs. "Peace, baby."

"I'm not a baby!" he snarls.

"Maybe not, but I call all my best friends 'baby'. So are you my friend or not?"

"Depends."

"Depends? Hmmm," Sim considers and makes a menacing face. "I think it's a lot better for your welfare to be on my side, baby."

"Okay," he agrees and he looks back at me.

"Hey, Jack," I assure him, "he calls me 'baby' too. I'm serious. I don't get any 'Officer, sir!' from him. Trust me on this."

He looks back at Sim. "Okay, baby," he says and Sim almost falls down laughing.

When he gets over it, he puts a hand on Jack's head and messes his dark hair.

"Gee, Sean, fucking good looking little rogue, isn't he? I didn't know they still made them this good. Jack? You can call me 'baby' or you can call me 'Dad'. Nice to meet you, honey."

He swings the front door open and waves me in and then he takes Jack's hand and walks him into the boardroom.

"Gentlemen?" he laughs with a proud smirk, "Good doctors, I'd like to introduce you to little Jack Mack. Jack, this is your uncle Dr. Mack and Dr. Jain. Jack, have a seat."

He pulls a chair out for Jack and pushes him in to the table. "Has he eaten, Sean? They don't have coffee at that age do they?"

"Milk please, baby." Jack corrects him.

"Hmmm. Milk, yeah." Sim goes to the kitchen for a glass of milk and nobody speaks while we wait for him. Jack slides slowly down his chair until all we can see are his blue eyes and the top of his head peeking nervously across the table.

Sim come back with the milk and scolds Jack gently. "Sit up, man! You're the guest of honor."

Jack wiggles back up and takes the glass with both hands.

"So what's the story, Sean?" Sim asks, sitting down again with his coffee. "You found him at my house?"

"Yeah. I spotted him a few times peeking in the window but he'd just run away when he saw me. He says he was afraid that his father was a cop. Crystal finally snuck up behind him and grabbed him and we sat him down to talk.

"His mother told him if anything ever happened to her that his father lived at the little beach house at the Point. She over-dosed a couple months ago on the Point Special, the trifecta blend: heroin, coke and meth.

"I wouldn't be surprised if she didn't score it from your house, from your personal chef, sorry to say."

"Ouch," Sim cringes. "Who the fuck was she?"

"Her name was Sandra. Does that ring a bell?"

"Crap, Sean, do you know how many babes named Sandy I've – uh?"

He stops himself short and looks at Jack. I wonder if he's going to have a change in vocabulary now. It could be amusing.

"Man, Jack baby," he sighs, "A junkie Mom? That's a lousy hand. I'm sorry, but I didn't know a thing."

He watches Jack sucking on the glass of milk.

"So, the million dollar question," Mack interjects, "What do you want to do about it now, Steven?"

"It's not a question, Mack," he laughs. "How could I kick a handsome little bastard like this back out on the street? He's obviously my boy. Put him up in the nurses' room with his new mother."

Jack's mouth drops open and he puts the glass down hard on the table. "I have a new mother, too?"

"Yeah, baby," Sim says. "You have a beautiful new mother. She's a nurse and she'll take very good care of you. Oh, man, she is going to love you, baby Jack!"

Jack bites his finger again and it looks like he's doing it to keep from crying. He sniffs and then smiles shyly. It's the first time I've ever seen him smile.

†

## S&M

"Any other Board business, Mr. President?" Mack asks with a sigh of relief.

"Yeah. I'm going to release the prisoner. Four days is long enough. I have a feeling she'll still be spending a lot of time in the nurses' room, but she's welcome back in the pool house. I don't want her fired.

"Also, I'd like to propose adding my little brother to the staff as Nat's assistant so she can start training him and put him to work. He's needs more focus than recreational sex."

"Your little brother?" Jain asks confused.

"Yeah. Psycho Kama David John. Right, Mack?"

"Yep, Jain," he nods. "We're claiming him. I believe he's Dad's kid. We might as well put him on the payroll."

"Fine with me," Jain laughs with a shrug. "We've got our differences settled now."

"Cool. Is it okay if I invite him to join us before we adjourn?"

Everyone agrees to wait while I get Dave. I find him laid out in the sun naked on a lounger by the pool, being massaged with sandalwood oil by

Nicky and Nat, with nothing covering his ass but a tea towel.

"Baby," I say poking his shoulder, "it's important. We need to see you in the boardroom."

"Awwww!" he moans.

Nat hands him a sarong and Nicky shows him how to wrap it and tie it. He's glowing with such a beautiful golden tan he looks like he just stepped off the beach in Bali.

"He doesn't like that, S&M," Nicky scolds me while she arranges the sarong on him. "Please don't call him baby any more."

"He's my baby, Nicky. I'll call him whatever I want. Right, Dave baby?"

"Absolutely, Nim," he laughs. "That's just your rules, Nicky."

"Yes, Psycho Sir," she concedes.

I put my arm around Dave's shoulder and start walking him back to the house.

"My fucking baby brother," I snarl at him and his eyes widen with surprise. "My fucking baby brother," I repeat just to hear the sound of it.

Mack stands up when we come in the room and shakes his hand and hugs him.

"Good to see you, little brother," he laughs looking him up and down in nothing but a sun tan and a saffron sarong. "Even if it's a bit more of you than I expected. We've been discussing your situation. Sit down. We need to talk."

Dave starts to pull out a chair and then he freezes when he notices Jack, nearly hidden under the table where he's slid down his chair again.

"Up, up, UP!" I command him. "Get up and give your Uncle Kama Dave a nice handshake. Behave yourself, son!"

"Uhm –What?" Dave stammers.

"Hah," I howl. "Welcome to my Universe, baby!"

Then I notice Dave is looking a little—traumatized.

"What, baby?" I beg him. "What's wrong?"

"You already have a son? I thought I—I thought you—and Brandy—I thought," he trails off.

Oh crap. I forgot about the adoption. I thought we all forgot about it. I step in front of him and put my hands on his shoulders, arms' length, just like we're going to spar, and I look deep in his eyes. Shit, they're already blurry with tears.

"Are you kicking me out, Nim?" he sniffs.

"Oh, no, no, no, baby! No. This is supposed to be good news. I mean, yes, I have a son or maybe a hundred, but that doesn't change us. I mean, no, I can't adopt you, but—I—"

I can see I'm just making a horrible tangle out of everything. Jack is completely invisible now hiding under the table with fright. Dave hasn't started bawling outright yet but there are tears streaming down. Mack interrupts and pushes the bourbon across the table to us.

"Dave. You're our brother," he says simply. "Calm down, man. Have a seat."

I pour us both a strong one.

"Half-brother we think," I add, "but that counts, baby. So I don't need to adopt you. You're my blood."

I give him a very intimate and knowing look that says a lot more than my words: there are going to be no more three-ways, brother.

He sniffs, then snorts some whiskey and starts to relax. Mack kicks off his shoes and puts his feet up on the boardroom table and Dave starts laughing.

"Brothers?" he wonders.

"Yeah well, we can do DNA tests but I think it's about as unnecessary as testing this one," Mack laughs pointing under the table.

"We want to talk to you about joining the staff, brother, working as Nat's apprentice. You may be an orphan but your father was a very rich man. Once your probation is over, we can talk about making you a full partner in the business."

Dave is speechless with joy. He looks from one face to another, from Jain's broad smile, to Sean's amused pride, to Mack's brotherly love. Then suddenly he looks down startled and confused.

"What the fuck?" he swears. "The little bastard punched me!"

Jack crawls out from under the table next to Dave and growls in his little childish voice, "Are you going to shake my hand or punch me, baby?"

Dave shakes his hand in a daze and Jack asks him sweetly, "Why are you dressed like a girl, Uncle?"

"Jack, don't be a little scrap of shit," I warn him. "That's how famous surfers dress. Show your uncle some respect."

"Uh, is he famous?" Jack asks respectfully.

"He's very famous," I exaggerate a little bit. "He won the Point Guard surf challenge."

Dave beams with pride. We adjourn the meeting and Sean thanks me profusely. I'm not sure why. I hope he doesn't start rounding up every nine-year old street kid who looks like me now.

"Look, man," he consoles me. "There may be a lot of them out there but they could already be in good hands, in good homes, adopted and cared for. This guy just had a bad turn of events. Or maybe a good turn of events now."

I take Jack's hand and put an arm around Kama Dave's shoulders and walk them out into the sunshine.

"So, Kamadev brother, do you want to go back to your slaves or do want to go see your, um—sister-in-law with me?"

He snorts. "Oh. With you, Nim!"

When we walk past the pool, Jack squeezes my hand nervously as all the heads turn. Nicky would know who the little scrap is since she saw all the letters to the newspaper. Nat would probably guess. There's eternal time enough to let them gossip.

But nothing's going to come between me and Dave. Not women. Not children. Especially not women I vow, remembering how happy he was watching her making love to me. Shit, Nicky isn't just my girlfriend now. She's my sister.

†

BRANDY

Sim leaves me at 10 in the morning. I've got three more days locked up here but I'm starting to have a little hope. He was with me and in me all night and—although he wouldn't let me touch him—it was the weirdest sweetest sex I've ever experienced. He kept his hands firm around my wrists like human shackles but he held me close.

When he leaves, I get down on the floor again to play with the puzzle. The floor feels solid and grounding. The puzzle is immense and I remember picking it out for Kamadev because I thought it was complex enough to keep him out of the deep end of trouble. Now it's my therapy, keeping me occupied.

I love Dave almost as much as I love Sim, but differently. I think I need to love Sim more along those lines, as a soul mate instead of a sex god. Or a mixture of the two would work.

It's nearly one o'clock now and I'm thinking about lunch. The puzzle is nearly halfway finished and it's enticing me with the image of the peaceful waterfalls and deep pools littered with flowers.

I hear a timid tap on the door but I don't get up to answer. I just call out 'Come in!' expecting maybe Sunny. The door opens a crack and a little boy slips through shyly. He stares at me but then he sees the puzzle and marvels.

"Ooohhh!" he barely whispers. He walks over and bends down for a good look and then he walks around me. "Ooohhh. What is it? It's a broken picture!"

While he devours the puzzle with his eyes, I eat him alive with mine. He looks like a little man, like Sim and Dave both, the most beautiful boy I've ever seen. He's dressed in brand new clothing, stiff little jeans and a dark blue child's t-shirt that says "Property of the Point Guard" with the police logo.

"Who are you?" I finally manage.

"I'm Jack, baby. I'm looking for my mom."

"Who's your mother," I wonder.

"Um, she's a beautiful nurse. I don't know," he says biting down on the side of his first finger with a helpless look back at the door.

The door opens wide and Sim and Dave are standing there laughing. I suppose it's some kind of trick they're playing on me.

"The bad news, Brandy," Sim begins seriously, "is this little scrap is going to need your shitty little bed. So you've got to go, honey. He's too old to sleep with you."

"I don't want to go, Sim," I beg. "I'm going to behave. I promise."

"I mean it's time to go home, Bran," he purrs. "The herb garden is looking like shit. You're free to come and go as you like."

I'm so confused now I want to cry but instead I pick up a piece of the puzzle and give it to Jack.

"Nah, it's too hard," he moans. "It's trouble."

I point to the space where it clearly goes and watch as he turns it this way and that before he figures it out. He laughs and looks at Sim with delight.

"Good job, baby," Sim smiles and sits on the floor with us. Dave gets down and picks up another piece and starts searching for its spot while Jack watches him carefully. I don't need to do the math. Dave is 21 and he was a virgin anyway.

Sim is just staring at me curiously.

"Good-looking little scrap isn't he?" he finally snorts. "It is what it is, Brandy. Youthful indiscretion. Do you think you could—?"

"Take care of him? He's yours?"

Sim nods.

"My greatest treasure!"

I know he doesn't want me to touch him but this is not about sex. I throw myself into his arms and kiss his cheeks, his neck, his forehead, his nose, his mouth. I kiss everything above the shoulder line and he seems delighted with it.

"Brandy. Good. Enough!" he finally orders.

Jack is watching the display of affection with amusement.

"Awww," he smiles. "Is she my mother?"

"Yes, baby Jack," Sim laughs. "She's yours—if you don't mind sharing with your Uncle Kama Dave."

†

DJ

"A kid that age needs a mother much more than a father, don't you think?"

Nim sounds like he's trying to convince himself more than me as we walk back to the pool. We left Jack with Brandy so we could finish up our business with the pool slaves.

"When you were 15 what you needed was a father but you wanted a mother. You followed Nicky around like a puppy. But at 9, he's missing his mom, not me. He doesn't even know me."

I remember Nim didn't have a father or a mother since he was 13. I'll bet he was missing them both. All he had was a brother. But I just nod as he continues.

"I've learned that the best way to keep someone out of trouble is to give them someone else to supervise, man. Jack will keep Brandy out of trouble so I can concentrate on my dharma."

"Which is?" I ask innocently, even though I know.

"Turning all the lights on," he laughs. "But it's a tough job so I need a massage first."

Nat and Nicky are horsing around in the water trying to drown Prince and he's hysterical with joy.

"Who's in charge here?" Nim roars. "We've got business. Out, out, OUT!"

He points to one of the lawn loungers for me and starts stripping while he barks orders.

"Prince, I need something special for dinner tonight for ten. What do you suggest?"

"How does veggie lasagna sound?" Prince asks averting his eyes from his naked boss. "And there's quite a bit of leftover crab. Crab Louis salad with sangria blanca and garlic bread."

"Fine. Get going. Make sure there's a lot of milk and cookies too."

"Nat?" He lies face down on one of the loungers and expects her to read his mind.

"No problem, boss," she says pouring the sweet oil on his back. "The scars are looking very nice now. How's the pain?"

He roars with laughter. "Is that really what's on your mind, Nat? The kid is mine. I'm keeping him. His name is Jack. He's nine years old and Brandy is taking care of him."

Nicky groans.

"Nick, get over it," he continues. "You can't adopt him. Nat, I want you to take Kama Dave on as your apprentice."

"Sure boss. What do you want him to do?"

"Inventory, orders, lab maintenance, laundry, flower arrangements, whatever you need. I want him to learn the business. Teach him all about the medicinals. He's training to be a partner."

Then he just shuts up and sighs while Nat works on him. All the lights are coming back on except one.

"Nim?" I remind him.

"I love you, man," he laughs. "Oh, yeah, that. Nicky, you're going to have to stop grabbing my ass. You're married to my brother. Behave yourself, sister."

I hold my breath to see if Nicky is going to scream or go crazy, but she doesn't make a sound. I think that might be more dangerous than anything. I look at her for a clue but she's busy inspecting her fingernails.

No one says a word for a long time. Nat keeps massaging. When she finishes with his feet, Nim finally instructs, "Dave? When were you thinking you'd like to start working?"

"Um—any time. Now?"

"That sounds like a very good plan for you, brother. I'll see you at dinner."

I look at Nat and she nods her head yes, wipes the oil off her hands on a towel and holds her hand out to me in Gyan mudra, the gesture of wisdom and learning.

I smile at her and get up. We've been dismissed.

†

NICK

I'm speechless. S&M waits without a word until Dave and Nat are out of sight and then he gets up from the lounger naked and sits cross-legged on the grass at my feet.

My god, he's laughing at me, not right out loud, but I can see it in his expression. I run my eyes over every inch of him with hunger and adoration. For nearly six years he's been my teacher, my protector, my boyfriend, my slave, but never my lover until a few nights ago. Now he says he's my husband's brother. It couldn't get any more complicated.

I'm somehow hoping for operating instructions, some kind of manual. Or maybe I'm waiting for him to tell me it's all a joke. Instead he points to the grass in front of him, inviting me to sit on the ground.

"How's my beautiful brother been behaving?" he asks kindly. "I haven't seen you since the picnic."

I think about what's gone on since then: a beautiful night alone in the forest with Dave, then the jealous rivalry building up in the gym, the fight in front of Jain, the dice game, how I thought I had beaten him and won everything he owned until he had me on my knees, under his thumb with his psycho sex.

"He's insane, S&M," is all I can say. "He's totally psychotic."

"You love him," he adds and it's not a question.

"Yes. Yes, I do. I love him very much. But I can't control him," I whine. I watch his face shining with joy and amusement. "Were you the one who taught him how to dance like that?"

"A little token of my affection for you, Nicky. I knew it would amuse you. You will never tire of him. He will keep you happy for the rest of your life."

I feel a tug at my heart. I know he's right but I—I...

"Shit, S&M. I love you. I love you! I love you so much it's painful." I'd like to bite him right now and make him gasp with pleasure. I'd like to see him on his knees.

"I love you too, sweetheart," he admits. "I've always loved you, Nicky. And I get off on your adoration."

"Then why, why have you pushed me away for all these years? Why not you and I, baby? And you married—a nurse for god's sake! You don't even know her!"

He laughs softly.

"I've got some pretty good reasons, Nick," he explains. "You say it's painful how much you love me. Multiply that by a hundred. We could hurt each other very badly, honey. We could completely destroy each other and everybody else around us, everyone we love. You're too much, baby, too much for me. I've got a lot of baggage and issues. I needed to start over from scratch and work out all my bad karma.

"Kamadev is beyond that. He's spotless, inviolable, dispassionate, enlightened. You can't hurt him. Trust me, honey, you need a psychotic boy, someone you can't drive mad!"

I can't believe what he's saying. He loves me too much to be my lover! I feel the heat rising up my spine and I want to crush him and beat some sense into him. Who is crazy now?

"If you think trying to control Kamadev is hard, honey, imagine what a horrible torture it would be for you to try to control Shiva. Aw, Nicky, I love you too much to do that to you. It would kill you.

"It's a lot easier for me to break in someone who doesn't know me, someone who isn't bent on controlling me. Brandy is a better student, sorry to say. She tried to control me too but she's already starting to cave in."

"So I'm back to being like a sister? Even after that—night? God, S&M, how do I just forget about that?"

"You don't forget about it. You enjoy it. Just like Nat will never forget taking Kamadev's virginity. But you just don't get attached to it. You enjoy the experience and let it go."

"Nat?!?" I spew. "She what?"

"Sorry, I thought you knew. She was so infatuated with him she had to have a taste. Once was enough. It was enough for both of them. She got over her desire and he learned how to, um—handle a goddess like you.

"Freedom comes from letting go of all your attachments. Dispassion, vairagya. You know these things, Nicky. I'm not going anywhere but you can't have me."

"Fuck." I hate to use that kind of language, but it's what he understands. "I'm like a sister again."

I wish he weren't so beautiful. I look at him like that perfect piece of cake I'm not allowed to taste. But I have tasted it. I'm just not allowed to have seconds.

"Not *like* a sister, beautiful. You *are* my sister. We're very sure Dave is our brother. I'm not sleeping with *him* again either!" he laughs nervously.

"And you can't adopt little scrappy Jack because he's already your nephew. Your family is just getting bigger, Nicky. Mack is your brother now and Brandy is your sister so maybe you can quit hating her a little, unless that's how sisters like to treat each other."

And I thought it couldn't get any more complicated! Whew! But he loves me. I can see it in his eyes. He loves me very much. Maybe we can still play. I wonder if it will ever be enough for me again.

I look over at his little pile of clothing, the fringe leather belt looped over his pants. He reads my mind.

"Not now, honey. Some other time." When I sneer at him, he quickly changes the subject.

"Man, Nicky!" he roars. "You should've seen Dave's face when he first saw Jack. It was like he spotted a rat in the kitchen cupboard. I swear I saw murder in his eyes just for a second, as if the kid was going to take his place. It's a good thing he's my brother. I think he loves me even more than you do!"

"Hang on, S&M," I suddenly realize. "Dave's going to be working with Nat now and she – oh, no!"

"Jealousy doesn't become you, Nicky. They got over it long before you got here. And Jain has made a lasting impression on him."

He gets up and gets dressed again and I feast on the show. He likes the adoration and I don't mind admiring him. As he watches me openly devouring him he laughs.

"Insatiable Kali! You impossible ravenous beast! At least I have a chance of containing my wife."

"Containing her?" I hiss. "That's just sick, S&M. Don't you want a soul mate?"

He looks at me like I'm mad. "You *are* my soul mate. You are *all* my soul mates. Every last one of you, from Mack to Jack. All of you are mine!"

He ties the belt on with a big grin, obviously relishing the effect he's having on me. And then he looks over his shoulder, back at the pool house and then over at the Fire House and his smile turns from amusement to a scorching sear.

"It's been a wild day," he confesses. "I might have enough time before dinner—to take a half dozen or so—just for my brother you know. Your place or mine, honey?"

†

## JACK

My father is like the king. My new mother said he is the President of all the houses on the top of the mountain, all three houses. The big house where I have my own new bedroom is called the Ice House because it has Intensive Care Emergency like a hospital. My Uncle Mack is a doctor. He lives there with a beautiful nurse, Sunny but they are not married.

The house next door is called the Fire House. My father named it after the Sun. It has Dr. Jain, his wife Nat, my Uncle Kama Dave with Aunt Nicky and Prince our chef. That is a very organized house with so many people. I can have anything I want to eat if I ask Prince to fix it. Prince is only twice my age so I like him very much.

My father who is the King of everything up here has his own house behind the pool called the Pool House. It is very, very small with only a tiny little room, a little kitchen and a shower bathroom, but it has a huge private deck above the tops of the forest trees, above the clouds. This is where my father lives with my new mother, but he says I am too old to sleep with them so I have my own room.

My mother says I have some rules and I like having rules because my old mother had none at all. Now she's dead and that's probably why. I think I like rules and order.

My rules are: don't go into the forest alone. Don't go in the pool alone. Don't leave the Ice House unless I tell someone where I'm going. My new room has a telephone with a lot of buttons and I can call any of the houses with it.

Mother says the reason the police officer is living in my father's beach house is because they work for him to protect all his friends. She says the police are our friends and they took care of my father when he was very hurt.

My old mother was afraid of the police and no one took care of her when she was hurt. I'm very lucky and safe here with such a big family and doctors and nurses and friendly police. I will follow the rules very carefully.

Mother plays with me on the floor with the puzzle in my new room. She asks if I want a bath before dinner but Crystal cleaned me up very nice before I came here and gave me nice new clothes and shoes. I even have real pajamas now.

I take the shoes off because my father doesn't wear them, but Mother says I should keep my shirt on for dinner. Dad and Uncle Kama Dave don't wear shirts. Mother says it's because they are too beautiful. And I can see they have lots of good muscles.

I'm too little for muscles yet, so I will wear my new Point Guard shirt for dinner. It's a very nice new shirt and Mother says it's more polite. When I get muscles I might not have to be so polite.

†

## S&M

Really, what do I care? It's no skin off my back. She's pretty careful about that. She's such a hungry girl that it doesn't bother me at all to play with her. In fact it's amusing to see how worked up Nicky can get over a little roughhouse. She craves it but little brother Kama Dave is really only interested in more esoteric practices. Sri Kamadev would much rather make love than war.

It's two sides of the same coin to me: pleasure and pain, desire and aversion, the cause of all suffering in the world. None of it sucks me in.

Playing with her strengthens my equanimity. If you look equanimity up in the dictionary, you will see a picture of me grinning back at you. Equanimity, *upeksha,* is one of the divine virtues, the 'four immeasurables'.

If it keeps her satisfied and spares my brother from a good thrashing, it's feeding the other three virtues simultaneously: kindness, compassion and the enjoyment of other peoples' joy.

I take her back to the pool house out on the deck. It's been a warm afternoon and the scent of the jasmine dripping from the rafters is sensuous and seductive. Keep it cool, I remind myself. No matter how heated she gets, it's just therapy. She can save the rest for Kama Dave.

And hot she is, the red-hot green-eyed serpent goddess of the mountains and the seven seas. Hotter than Kali trampling Shiva under her heels after she bites the heads off every man in sight and tears off their arms. Hot enough to bring almost any man to his knees. Which is why she's so much fun to play with. I will not let her crush me.

I hand her my fringed belt and smirk into her emerald eyes, just turning up the heat—and she ignites. My sole intention is to simply defuse her. I could do it with one hand tied behind my back blindfolded. I could do it even easier handcuffed.

"Hands on the wall," she commands.

But when I turn my back on her and lean into the wall, nothing happens. I turn my head and grin at her but she looks grave and grim as if she's lost her appetite. She puts her hands on my bare back and smooths it out like a silk sheet and then she takes her hands lower and—fuck.

She starts to swear softly and terribly, running her hands over my gunshot scars. She's seen it all before. I've been running around half naked since she's been here. But now she seems to really see it, to feel it.

"I will kill the fuckers who did this, S&M!" she swears. "I'll tear their fingers off one by one and cut their tongues off."

"Probably not," I take my hands off the wall and turn around to look in her eyes. "They're serving life prison terms. You probably won't have the opportunity."

All the light has gone out of her eyes and nearly all the fun has been extinguished. I don't like the looks of it.

"You know," I warn her, "pity sucks. Compassion is pretty sweet but pity sucks the joy out of everything. You don't enjoy adding pain to injury. What you love is assaulting power—putting strength to the test.

"Admit it. You can't play if I'm hurt. Get over it, sister. I think the scars look pretty damn powerful."

She looks down at the damage on my belly, a little nicer than the piecework puzzle on my back, and I can see her eyes smoking with fury.

"It doesn't hurt in the least bit," I lie. "Are you going to play with me or what, Nicky? I haven't got all day."

She huffs and then smiles weakly. Aw, this is going to be like walking on cake for me today. She's caving in too. I turn my back on her again and put my hands up on the wall, flex my back and then wiggle my ass a little to wake her up.

Wham!#! That does it. She unleashes the Furies on me, the three goddesses of vengeance: Murder, Jealousy and Anger. I feel the smack and hear the crack. Game On. 1-0.

"That one is for sleeping with your nurse!" she hisses. I hear her breathing hard through her nose and she takes a second shot over my right shoulder.

"That one is for being celibate for seven years!"

The count is 2 and 0. I wonder, in all fairness, how I can be accused of being a slut and a celibate at the same time, but fury has no logic.

The third strike is a charmer and it comes down with coarse brutality. "That one is for abandoning a hundred beautiful little bastards!"

Ouch. Ooooh, yeah, I deserve that one.

"Do that one again, Nicky," I advise her and she whacks me into next week, four to nothing.

"Maybe I should give you a hundred," she sneers. "Brother!" she spits the word out like it tastes terrible.

"Nah, six is good enough, honey," I laugh.

She's giving me some serious pain and I'm paying attention to the way it radiates downward, mainly to my feet, through the wooden deck boards and out into space. The pain rolls off my skin like rainwater and it feels oddly cleansing.

I don't suppose lashing number five should come as any surprise to me but she digs deep for it.

"That one is for letting Nat put her hands on my beautiful boy!"

And though she prides herself in never leaving a mark or a trace of her handiwork, that one might have gone overboard. She stops and puts her hand on my back to check for any damage and then I hear her gasp.

I look over my shoulder and she's staring at Brandy who apparently just came quietly through the kitchen door with my little boy's hand in hers. Brandy is watching with a mixture of shock and awe and Jack looks amazed.

"Why are you hitting my father?" he wonders.

Without thinking twice Nick turns and says sweetly, "Because he is so big and strong, Jack. I'm just testing him and checking to make sure he is still bulletproof."

"How is he?" Jack asks.

"Absolutely indestructible," she smiles. "He has a perfect unbreakable warranty."

"That's why he's the King, baby," Jack laughs.

†

## NAT

"Whadya got in there?" I remember him teasing the first time I showed Kama Dave my little lab. He was still completely stoned on narcotics and I'm sure his curiosity about the medicinals in the cabinets arose from anything that's locked up.

This time he brings experiential knowledge to the table and I can really start teaching him. I'm honored to have a new student and I'm grateful that he's learning to trust me again as a friend and teacher.

We start by unlocking everything and taking all the vials off the shelves, arranging them on the counter and taking inventory. He works diligently and meticulously and I encourage him to open and inhale anything that interests him.

I know which ones attract him and some are already old his favorites, particularly the sedatives, meditatives and aphrodisiacs. Jasmine, sandalwood and lotus are the ones he likes to call his 'love oils'. I don't need to teach him anything more about those!

I introduce him to cinnamon first to broaden his knowledge. It's much more than an aphrodisiac; it works as an astringent, antibacterial, antiseptic and disinfectant. It's very rare in botantical medicine to find a plant that isn't complex and multi-talented in its gifts to humanity.

I also point out to him that his love oils have other very nice applications. Jasmine and sandalwood, for example are also relaxing and healing to the skin like lavender.

Lavender is a great extract for him to start his studies because of its complex benefits. Along with helichrysum, it's also one of the most important oils I have for working with Sim's scars and wound healing.

I open a vial of high altitude French lavender and a vial of Kashmir lavender from the Himalayan foothills and let him compare the two. Both are exquisite oils, calming, spiritually uplifting and clarifying to the mind.

He likes the Kashmir oil best so I decide to teach him how to create a special blend for a specific application.

"How do think your little nephew is feeling right now in a completely new strange family?" I ask.

"He looked scared to death, Nat, like he wanted to disappear."

"Imagine you were trying to create something nice for a frightened child. You don't want love oils, you don't need wound care, you just want something to create a sense of calm and safety. Lavender is a wonderful place to begin."

I give him a little shot glass to mix in and suggest a few other synergistic ingredients. Cedar is lovely for stress and anxiety. Camomile is relaxing without causing any depressant effects, especially beneficial for children.

"You can use more or less of any of the oils to your liking, but I suggest you start with equal amounts and then adjust it."

He smiles shyly and his eyes sparkle like a mad scientist as he pours a half dozen drops of lavender, then sniffs the cedar and adds six drops, stirring the blend with a little glass rod. Then he does the same with the camomile and nods, holding it out to me.

"Very nice!" he says with pride. "Very balanced. I like the lavender best though. Can I?"

"Absolutely. Add a few more drops of lavender and see if you like it better."

When he's happy with the blend he breaks out a big grin and pours the oil into a fresh bottle. We label it 'Rx Jack'.

"This is what you did for me, Nat, isn't it? When I was sick. You made something to calm me down."

"Yeah," I laugh, "It was a whole lot stronger than this though! You were a raging lunatic junkie when you got here. I made a blend to deal with wild prana, traumatic shock and addiction. The idea is to make something specific to create the desired effect you want."

He sniffs the little bottle with his new blend, first on the left side and then on the right. His eyes are soft and calm and thoughtful now.

"What would you make for a very jealous girl? A very ravenous, hungry wild girl? I think she's getting too many love oils."

"Oh! Nicky!" I laugh. "That's pretty easy. She's off the charts with jealousy. She's jealous of me and Brandy and Rick and Sim and Jack and you and, God bless her, I think she's even jealous of herself!

"Jealousy is a sign of Pitta imbalance: too much heat. She definitely doesn't need more aphrodisiacs! I think you'll like what this does."

I put the lavender in front of him again.

"The same blend you made for Jack would be nice for her, but let's make a special Wild Woman blend for Nicky."

Next to the Lavender, I put a vial of Rose Geranium.

"For wellbeing and sensuality, very uplifting and supportive for the female endocrine system," I wink at him.

"And this one, Rhu Khus, the 'Oil of Tranquility'. You can probably add a little of that to Jack's blend as well, just to ground everything else.

"A little tranquility goes a long way," I tease him. "Why don't you make a really big batch of that one? I'll bet Brandy could use a little bit, too."

†

## BRANDY

Poor baby. What have we brought him into? He watches his father being thrashed by that psycho bitch and he thinks it's cool; he's impressed. This is not good.

I turn around to get him the hell out of here but Sim pulls up a yoga mat and motions for me to sit.

"What?" he says seriously, slightly offended. "What? There's nothing wrong with it."

I look at Nicky and she seems transformed. I expect to see her in a jealous rage, but she's calm and beneficent. And she's lusting after little Jack like he's a precious diamond.

"Sweet sister," she purrs. "I've just learned we are family—you and me, Dave, Mack, S&M and Jack. I'm sorry for being such a jealous girl. But I think you can understand. My sweet brother is worth his weight in heartache."

Sim pats her on her head and then puts a hand around her back whispering loud enough for me to hear.

"I'll take a rain check on number six. Get lost, sweet sister."

And she's gone.

I don't know where to begin. I'm shocked and alienated from Sim, at a distance like I'm looking at him through the wrong end of binoculars. Little Jack sits next to me on the mat and Sim just sits in front of us, carrying on as if no one has missed a beat.

"Oooh, Jack," he laughs. "Do you know how to swim, honey? Can you surf?"

Jack smiles and shakes his head.

"Dog paddle. I won't drown but it's not good," he says.

"Cool. We'll teach you. Your Mom can help."

Jack obviously adores him. Sim worries me terribly but I'm helplessly under his spell too. I'm surprised that he's taking fatherhood so calmly. But like the enlightened being he is, he shifts gears so fast my head spins.

"Jack," he starts, "straighten up, buddy. Nice and relaxed, legs crossed but let your spine rise. Be tall, little scrap."

Jack sits in a beautiful easy pose and rises up his spine as much as a nine year old can.

"I'm going to start by teaching you mudras, baby," Sim continues. "Mudras are little hand signals that communicate ideas and energy—outward and inward.

He sticks his hand out with the middle finger extended in the 'fuck you' gesture.

"That one? Seen that?"

Jack laughs.

"That's not nice. It's not yoga. How about this one?" He shows him the peace sign.

"Mmm, peace baby," Jack hums with pleasure.

"Yes, and it comes from a yoga mudra, the two rivers of prana that run along your spine, fire and ice, the sun and the moon combining to create peace and balance.

"This one is my favorite, Ahimsa. It means 'No harm. Nothing to fear'." He holds his palm up like the teaching Buddha.

"And this one, Gyan mudra is very sweet for you. It looks like the 'okay' sign. What it means is wisdom and what it does is make you feel calm and centered. First finger and thumb create a circle and the other three fingers are counting your blessings.

"Here's a nice little practice for you, buddy. Start just like that with the thumb on the first finger, then on the second finger, third finger, little finger. The rest, the meaning, comes later but that should calm you down for now, baby."

Jack is in awe of him and drinks in the attention like a boy dying of thirst. I watch him playing with the finger positions and smiling happily to himself.

"Good boy," Sim laughs. "Do you feel safe to go out and play by yourself before dinner?"

"I have my rules, Dad baby," Jack says. "Don't go in the forest or the pool alone. Don't go out of the Ice House unless I tell someone."

"Cool," he says. "I'd like to talk to your mother. You're free to play outside for an hour. Then I'll come and get you for a special dinner in your honor at the Fire House. Got it?

Jack nods respectfully and gets to his feet. He flashes Sim the 'okay' gyan mudra with a beautiful shy smile and takes off.

When he's gone, Sim snarls at me like he's about to bite my head off. I squirm under his ice blue gaze.

"And?" he begins. "Did you have any questions for me?"

I want to be so careful not to offend him, so cautious and politically correct, but the situation is wild. I don't want to be sent away again. I'm afraid the next time will be the last time.

"That, uh—stuff with Nicky," I stammer, "does that turn you on?"

He throws his head back and roars with laughter.

"Oh, my beautiful sweet Brandy, my most beautiful student, you don't have a clue. You still don't know me in the least bit.

"*Everything* turns me on. Everything that *moves* turns me on!"

He leans forward onto his hands and crawls on hands and knees towards me putting his face into mine like a big cat with a mad Cheshire smile.

"Everything!" he growls.

"And, uh—," I continue, "I wonder if I should learn how to do that? To whip you. Do you like that?"

"Silly girl," he laughs. "Of course not. I could care less about that. She likes it and Dave doesn't. I just enjoy the lila, the play. I'd rather play at something you like.

"Puzzles? Books? Dice? Preferably not hypodermic needles. What do you like to play, Brandy?"

He's just sucked all of the oxygen out of the atmosphere on the deck. I can't breathe. What do I like? Oh, holy honey, I want him more than anything.

"You," I groan. "I want to play with you."

His smile fades and I see tears rising in his eyes as he sits back on his heels seriously.

"I thought you were learning, Brandy," he sighs. "I'm not a game, sugar. I'm not a toy."

†

S&M

Damn it, I'm *very* aroused but I can't just cave in. She was very, very bad, the trifecta of bad with the handcuffs, drugs and rape. If I give in now, I'm lost. I'm not willing to settle for a fuck; I want love to the highest power.

My wife hangs her head at my rejection and watches the deck carefully. That's good. Don't talk to me, don't look at me, and don't touch me. These are my rules and the dice are loaded.

"Speaking of games," I sneer sweetly, "What the fuck did you do with my handcuffs?"

She looks up, not at me, but over the top of the trees and points.

"Down there," she whispers. "I was afraid. I threw them off the deck. Somewhere down there."

"You should be afraid, sweetheart. That was very, very bad."

"I know, Sim. I'm sorry."

"Well at least we've got a new game to play now, a treasure hunt. Let's go."

I take her hand and help her to her feet. I want to pull her into my arms and hold her and take away her fear, but I need to teach her. I need to trust her again.

When we leave the pool house, Jack is sitting on the lawn engrossed in some child's play. We walk around the side of the house towards the forest trail without saying a word. After a minute I reach out and hold her hand.

"Shit. They're not just any handcuffs," I tease her. "Dave was arrested in those."

They've seen a lot of nicer action as well but I leave the rest to her imagination as we walk deeper into the forest down below the deck. I can think of more good times than bad that we had with my toy. I slip an arm around her waist and she holds her breath.

"Breathe!" I laugh. "Remember what Kamadev taught you. This is only the frosting, sugar."

She laughs nervously but I have to let go of her because the mountainside falls away so steeply behind the house as we cut away from the main trail. The brush is dense and the task of finding anything down here is daunting. Dropping something off the deck is as good as launching it into orbit.

The tall grasses are knee high. I find a couple of large shards from the potted plants that I threw off the deck in a rage months ago, a mutilated chair and a piece of the massage table that is still stuck up in the tree top.

"Oh, those were the days," I laugh. "Remember Dave keeping us awake crying all night?"

"Remember how frightened he was of Nat?" she adds. "She wasn't even allowed upstairs. I hope I—I hope we can look back on this and laugh. I mean you loved those handcuffs. I hope I didn't ruin them for you."

I give up looking and sit down in the tall grass and stare at her. She is so nervous and perfectly obedient now I'm ready to forget everything. I hold my hand out and she comes over and sits on my lap, wrapping her legs around my waist.

"Just this," I instruct. "Nothing more. Maybe this, too," I give her a small kiss on her mouth. "Nothing more."

I watch her chocolate brown eyes melt in the late afternoon sunshine into liquid gold. What is she hiding in there behind those dark windows? I start singing softly to her, lam, vam, ram, yam, ham, aum, ah oh ooh mmm, and sweet orgasms start racing through me.

Nothing more. Maybe just this too, this uh—ahum—and then I just bury my tongue in her mouth and crush her in my arms. I'm lost and it's only just a kiss accompanied by fully clothed full body orgasms jolting through my veins like a fire hose pumping full blast.

When it finally subsides, I lie back on the forest floor and pull her down in my arms and rock her. I really didn't see that coming, but it feels nice and sweet and safe lying here in the tall grass.

She puts her mouth against my ear and whispers, "Are you positive you're not a toy? Possibly an adult toy?"

I roll over on top of her and pin her helplessly against the dirt. "I'll show you who the toy is," I snarl at her. And then a little gleam of metal catches my eye above her head: the head of the key still in the lock of my lost handcuffs nearly buried in the peat soil.

I pull them out of the dirt with a victory howl. Just as I'm getting set to restrain my helpless prisoner, I hear little whispering and laughter in the forest.

I freeze and listen putting my finger to my lips. Her eyes widen as she hears it too, a little voice somewhere in the forest above us. I pull her up to her feet and we start quietly back through the brush towards the trail.

On the side of the trail Jack is squatting down under a tree talking to someone invisible. He giggles and then, seeing us, he holds his palm up at arm's length. But clearly, from his body language, it's not intended as ahimsa, 'no fear'; it means 'stay back!'

"Son," I warn him, "what was the first rule your mother gave you?"

"I'm not in the forest alone, Dad," he explains. "I've got my little friend here showing me around."

He stands up lifting a copper red, white and black kingsnake in one of his hands, nearly as long as he is tall.

"This is my pal, Fang," he introduces the snake wrapping it around his shoulders. The snake rears his head at us in a polite greeting.

Brandy nearly goes down in a faint but she collects herself and grabs my arm, desperate to stay on her feet. It's going to be hard to get her to lie down in the grass again.

†

JACK

Fang is the most beautiful pet I've ever had. Uh – the only one ever. His skin is painted criss-crossed in red, orange, black and white and he is almost as big as me but much, much thinner. He is very friendly and very happy to be in the forest but when I show him to my mother she looks sick.

But my father takes him and wraps him around his own shoulders with a smile. They look so beautiful together, all wild and slinky.

"Can I keep him, Dad?" I beg. "He's my best friend in the world."

"You can't own him, Jack," he explains. "He belongs to all of us. He lives on the mountain. He would not be happy locked up in your room. But we can play with him as much as you want. He seems to like your company."

"Oooh," I moan. "But I want him in my new room."

"Nah, baby. We'll just come down here and play with him. He really likes the forest better. No shoes, no shirts, no rules. He's a kingsnake. He's in charge of the mountain."

"Like you?"

"Yeah, just the same. We'll come back tomorrow after breakfast and play with him. But now we've got a big dinner planned and believe me, honey, Fang would not enjoy it.

"If you really love him, let him be. He'll be here."

So I let my mother take my hand and Dad gives Fang a pretty kiss on the face and tucks him against a warm sandstone rock. We walk back up into the sunshine and leave my best friend alone in the forest and go off to the big dinner.

When we get to the Fire House, there are already a lot of people sitting around the big boardroom table but my father takes me through the kitchen into a little room which he says is his laboratory.

Uncle Kama Dave is in there with Aunt Nicky and Nat and they are all fighting. Well not exactly. Only Auntie Nicky is fighting. The rest are calm. Aunt Nicky is burning up words and hot sentences and poor Uncle Kama is trying to sweet talk her.

Dad breaks all of it up. He puts his arms around Nicky and holds her, heart to heart with her arms pinned against his chest.

"Sister," he hums. "What the fuck part of divine perfection is missing here, hmm?"

She beats on his heart with her fists and moans, "That. Bitch. Says. I'm. Jealous."

Dad just holds her and rocks her and waits. Nat nods at Dave and he starts to explain.

"Nim," he says proudly, "I mixed this beautiful oil for her and one for Jack. I told her it would help with sex-crazy jealousy and now she's furious at me.

"The one for Jack is for peace and safety. Maybe I should have started her with that."

"Nicky," my father scolds her, "Behave yourself. You can't argue with the truth. Why don't you give Dave a chance to show you what he's got for you?"

"Hmmmpf," Dave snorts. "I think I'd rather start with Jack."

He picks me up and sits me on the massage table and turns to Nat with a puzzled look.

"For someone that young I recommend the crown, forehead and heart," she advises. "Then dilute some into the carrier oil and massage his feet. But start with inhalation, okay?"

Uncle Dave lets me smell the bottle and it's very nice and soft smelling like the forest. He puts a drop on the top of my head, one between my eyebrows and one on my heart and then he starts to mix it up with another nice oil.

"So, Jack," he asks me while he stirs it up. "What have you been up to while I've been working?"

"I found a big kingsnake to be my friend!" I say. "Very nice and slinky."

He starts rubbing the oils into my feet and it feels so slippery and wonderful. Nicky is being very quiet now with Dad's arms around her watching me sweetly and so I smile back at her. She is the most beautiful lady I have ever seen with green eyes and golden brown hair.

I think how pretty Fang would look wrapped around her shoulders like a necklace. She winks at me and I laugh. She looks like a princess. I wonder why she isn't the queen.

"And I watched Aunt Nicky testing Dad," I explain. "He's fine. He has a warranty."

Uncle Dave looks up at her curiously.

"Testing?" he wonders.

"Yeah," I say. "With a belt. She's making sure he's still bulletproof."

Nat starts giggling very hard and has to sit down in a chair. Dave narrows his eyes and takes me off the table and points at Nicky.

"You, bad girl!" he commands. "It's your turn."

Dad takes his arms off Aunt Nicky and slaps her butt and she sits on the massage table with a frown.

"Come on, Jack. Nat," Dad says. "let's get out of here. And Dave brother, just do her feet or you'll miss dinner. You need to be there."

†

## MACK

It's a full house for dinner, all ten of us now. Sunny is helping Prince and apparently the plan to defend their kitchen fortress is to ply us with sangria blanca while they assemble the feast.

Everybody tries to take a sneak peek or a quick taste but Sunny throws them out just as quickly. The aromas of the lasagna and garlic bread are borderline torture but finally everything is assembled and they start bringing out crab louie salads, hot bread and more sangria.

Sim bangs on the lab door until Kama Dave and Nicky come out with their arms around each other. Then there's a scramble as Nicky insists on moving Jack over so she can sit between Sim and Jack. Dave makes Brandy move so he can sit across from Nicky and leer at her.

When they're settled I stand up and raise my glass.

"Ladies, gentlemen, friends, brothers, sisters, we're here to celebrate family. Please welcome my youngest brother, David John Dixon Mack and our recent arrival, Jack Mack."

Everyone cheers and toasts and then I turn to Dave and say, "What the hell am I supposed to call you now, little brother? Are you still going to use Nicky's last name or are you going to be a Mack?"

Dave gets to his feet and looks around the table and takes a big swig of the spicy wine and leers slyly at Nicky.

"I'm Kamadev Dixon, thanks," he laughs. "She owns me, brother. I wouldn't change a thing."

It's a good thing, I think. Nobody calls me David either, but that's my first name, after my father, so he would be the third David Mack if he was inclined.

"Cool," I say. "Welcome to the family. I'd also like to announce that Kama Dave is invited to join the Board of Directors when his six months probation is finished. In the meantime, he's apprenticing under Nat on Steven's staff—and still under house arrest.

"I'll let my other brother introduce the next guest of honor."

"What can I say?" Sim laughs. "This probably won't be the end of it. They're out there."

Then he looks over at Jack who's sliding down his chair again in embarrassment.

"What? What?" he growls. "Sit up! Why aren't you eating, man?"

"What the fuck is it, Dad?" Jack whines.

"Crab salad. It's rock'n'roll. Prince made it for you."

"What the fuck is crab, baby?" Jack moans.

"Oh, shit," Sim swears. "Try it. And don't say 'fuck' at the table until you're at least 12, okay?"

"Okay," Jack mumbles and pokes at the dish. Nicky leans over and squeezes a wedge of lemon on his salad and smiles at him. He stares at her as she puts a bit on his fork and puts it in her own mouth and winks. Then she feeds him a bite with the next forkful and he laughs.

"Nice, thank you!" he smiles at Nicky. "Delicious."

"Like I said," Steven laughs, "no DNA tests are required. He's already a ladies' man. Please welcome my son, Jack."

With the formalities settled, Prince and Sunny go back to the kitchen for the main course and the roar of the room escalates as pitchers of sangria disappear into thin air. The noise is punctuated by the arrival of trays of lasagna, more hot bread and refilled pitchers.

I take it easy on the wine. It's delicious, laced with fruit, brandy and prosecco; but I know it can be surreptitiously lethal so I switch to bourbon after the first toasts. I know bourbon like I know morphine. You get exactly what you pay for.

Steven seems delighted with the gross shift in his family arrangements and that makes me a little nervous. Mr. Equanimity is only a few deep breaths from grandiose delusionary disorder. He embraces a sudden strange young son, a schizophrenic brother, a sister-in-law girlfriend and a nymphomaniacal wife with the grace and submissive forbearance of a saint.

I want to keep an eye on him. On the sliding scale of manic depression, he's in the deep end of mania, howling with joy, whispering to his girl, leering at his wife, praising his son and just plain smirking at his new brother.

As much as I love to see my brother happy, I know him well enough to know there's a thin borderline between happiness and horror. I watch Brandy, such a sweet intelligent young woman, nervously watching him, bathed in love and lust but hopelessly intimidated by her husband.

After the food has been cleared, Prince serves an almond crème brulee and coffee for the adults and cookies with milk for Jack. Nicky trades her brulee for cookies and dips them lovingly in her coffee while Jack adores her.

"Fine, fine!" Steven barks, getting a little drunkenly to his feet when desserts are finished. "Let's have a toast to the women and the children! To the beautiful women, Brandy, Sunny, Nat and last but never the least, the goddess Nick.

"And to the children, Prince—yes, you baby are well under 21—and Jack.

"And now, the women and children are dismissed. Get lost, go home, go to bed and leave the men in peace. Good night, ladies and babies!"

A mixture of complaints and laughs go around the room, but the party breaks up. Prince and Sunny go back to the kitchen to clean up, Nicky and Brandy take Jack home to tuck him in with bedtime stories, and Nat kisses the crown of Jain's head and retreats to the bedroom.

What's left around the boardroom table is simply the future board: the President, CEO, CFO and our new apprentice. Steven, Jain, me and Kama Dave: the 'Boys'. The President and the apprentice are both clearly drunk and still pounding them back. I raise an eyebrow toward Jain but he smiles and raises his glass.

"Sometimes you've got to blow off a little steam, Mack," he laughs. "Sometimes it's the only cure for a train wreck."

Steven comes around the table and puts his arm around me and slurs, "Yer the bess brotha – 'cept this one, thas even betta, a new bess bro. An Jain Lover Boy, good as a bro. Ah love ya, Mack.

"I'd kiss ya all of ya but I'm not that kinda boy, brothas. Ahm in total—purr fect control."

And he breaks out laughing.

"Yeah, we all love you too, Sim," I say. "But I think you ought to get a little sleep. Time for the men to go home too."

"Ya think?" he looks surprised. "I'm jess now wakin up. Night's young. Stars and stuff."

"Look, I'll walk you home. Jain's going to bed."

"Oooh ya? Walk me?"

"Unless you need to have Jain carry you."

"Walk," he laughs.

I get up and take his arm, steadying him and we head out the back door, but Dave follows.

"Where you going, little brother?" I wonder. "You're already home, you live here. Go up to bed."

"Nah, Nick's not here. She's at your house with Jack. I'll walk Nim too and then walk Nicky home."

It sounds reasonable enough to me so the three of us start up the path towards my house. When we get to the gym though, Sim digs his heels in and stops.

"Dave?" he teases. "Night's young. Sparring?"

"Oh, yeah!" Dave snorts. "Sparring!"

"What?" I ask amazed. "Are you talking about fighting? I don't think that's a good idea right now."

"The bess idee, bro, drunken sparring, no pain!"

"Ah crap," I swear.

"Can't be stopped, Mack, night's young, stars and all. Women and children all gone."

He turns to Dave and pops him in the face. Dave howls with joy and smacks him back, then grabs Sim's shoulders to keep himself from keeling over. They both hit the pavement in unison.

They don't even bother trying to get to their feet. They just sit on the path laughing.

"Nim, ya got blood on ya," Dave laughs. "How bout me? Am I nice?"

Steven's nose is bleeding either from the smack or from hitting the ground with his face, impossible to tell. He looks up at me with a pathetic grin and begs, "Sofa? Please? Ahm given up now, brah."

I help him stumble over to the sofa and he crashes on it softly and sighs, "Ah stars. Good. Night."

Dave crawls after him and takes a seat, throwing an arm around his shoulders.

"I won, Nim. First blood, you loser!" he sneers.

"Look guys," I warn them. "You're on your own. Perfect control, my ass! Chill out and sober up. The night is young. Enjoy the light show."

I see Sunny coming up the path, finished cleaning the kitchen.

"Oh, beautiful Sunshine," I call out to her. "Perfect timing. Let me walk you home, darling."

†

DJ

Mack leaves us on the sofa and the whole Universe becomes brilliantly quiet. The Milky Way is already stunning and Nim starts singing milky blues lullabies to the stars.

"I can't quit you darlin', you are my heart's desire!"

He moans and slurs and howls with laughter.

"Uh uh! Oh ooo! Mmm hmmm!"

I look into his eyes and they are drunken with joy and sparkling with starlight. And then they go wide and curious and he hisses, “Shhhhh!”

I hear a door shut and voices and then I see Nicky walking home alone in the dark. We freeze and she walks past us without noticing there are two drunken brothers slouching on the sofa in the starlight staring at her.

We wait until she’s gone and we hear the door shut next door and then he starts to breathe again and sings in a whisper, “My one and only heart’s desire! Mmm hmmm!”

“Love her, Nim? My wife?” I whisper.

“Course, man,” he sighs. “Pain fully. My sister, shit! I don wanner, bro. Shores. She. Is. Yours. Save me, Kama. Protect me, man!”

“Love Bran?” I ask. “Ya gonna keep her or what?”

“Ya. Keeper. Keepin’er. Love, love’er. Crazy psycho nympho nurse! Oooh, not that psycha tick is bad, bru, can’t be stopped.”

He gets very quiet for a while and I suspect he’s doing the same thing as I am, watching the Universe spinning above him.

“Better go home, Kama bro,” he finally says. “Sleep with my sis so you don’t have bad dreams. None of this is gunna stop moving tonight. I can control—supervise the Universe. Go home.”

“Nah,” I say. “Night’s young. Stars and all. I’ll help ya supervise. Is zis fuckin boat a sleeper sofa?”

“Mmmm,” he purrs. He leans over to look for a latch under the side of the sofa and falls on his face. “Mmm, shit!”

I get up and drag him off to the side and lie on the ground on my belly feeling all around the bottom edges of the sofa and find the latch and – magic, it pops open. I unfold the poor old sofa into a lumpy old bed and then push Nim back up onto it.

"Fuggin deluxurioush," he moans. "The Ritz under a canopy o' galaxies."

And no sooner does he lie back and sigh on the deluxe lumpy sofa bed under the canopy of the night, he passes out with an awesome snore. I can't be bothered going home.

It's not the first time I've slept with him, but it's the best. I lie down next to my brother and listen to the gravelly snores serenade me like a lullaby. I watch the stars spin a web around us until my eyes are woven shut.

I dream I am falling out of the Milky Way like a shooting star and I hit the Earth with a big splash into an endless lake of milk. All around me cookies float like water lilies on the surface of the milk as I sink deeper and deeper into the darkness.

†

## NICK

For the first time since I've been at Sunrise, I wake up alone. My sweet boy never came home last night. Brandy and I walk little Jack home and we tell him stories until he falls asleep. Brandy tells him stories about monsters and heroes and I tell him the ones I learned from his father, the stories of the yogi gods and goddesses, Shiva and Kali and Parvati and Kamadev.

Nine years old is a complicated age. He looks like a little man but he's childishly insecure, starving for attention but worried he might be noticed. He reminds me a lot of his father, craving instructions and praise but determined to organize himself personally. Hmm, I laugh to myself. S&M

behaves like a confused pre-adolescent, how amusing.

Brandy and I have something in common now, someone other than S&M. I can't say we're friends yet, but I feel a little less jealous and a little more sympathetic to my—gulp—sister. At least she's never molested Dave; she's always treated him like his nurse, his mother, his sister, his friend.

Maybe Kamadev's wild woman anti-jealousy oils are working on me because I feel a little kinder. I crawl into bed and wait and wonder what happened to Dave but before I can speculate, the wine comes over me and I drift into sleep.

When daylight starts to creep over the mountaintop, I reach out for him and find an empty bed beside me. At first I feel anger rising but it quickly melts into concern. He was drunk when I left; maybe he's hurt.

No one is stirring downstairs. I walk out into the early morning and hear the first birds singing, even before the sun has risen. I'm thinking of checking the pool house but as I pass the gym, I see the boys passed out on the sofa, their arms wrapped around each other.

Now my concern explodes into the green-eyed monster of jealousy. How dare they sleep together without me! Do they really love each other more than they love me? I have every intention of waking them both up with a good sound thrashing, but as I get closer, my heart melts.

I love them both so much and they look so beautiful lying together dressed like matching book-ends, bare chested and barefoot in their leathers. S&M has a lot of dried blood on his face and Kama Dave has a little spit dripping on the fist he's sucking. They look like innocent little ruffians escaped from juvenile hall.

I remember S&M patiently teaching me the verses from Hafiz:

*Even after all this time*
*the Sun never says to the Earth*
*'you owe me'*
*Look what happens with a love like that.*
*It lights the whole sky!*

Just at that moment, the sun rises over the forest and I feel my heart heating up. I feel a bottomless love beyond sex, beyond ownership, and I know that's exactly how they love each other, a love like the Sun, lighting up the whole sky, a love that shines unconditionally without losing any of its intensity or fervor.

Instead of thrashing them, I go quietly back to the Fire House to get them coffee and croissants.

†

DJ

Nim wakes me up with a big snort and a kick but when I open my eyes he's in deep dreams, humming with pleasure. I don't move. I really can't move without waking him because I'm all tangled up with him, his arm wrapped around my neck.

I watch and wait. It's very fun to watch and I have to try very hard to keep from laughing. I bite my tongue and just grin. He's half singing, half humming like he did last night, "Oh ooh, Mmm hmm, OoHm, Om!"

Little jolts of pleasure are running through him and I hear him gasp between the Oms. The whole Universe is coming this morning and Nim is leading the parade. I even get a couple contact orgasms from him through my throat chakra.

Nim was wasted last night. I was drunk but he was brutally hammered. Before he passed out, he said he's in love with my wife. Fine with me. Who wouldn't love her? But he also asked me to protect him from her.

He loves Brandy, too. He said Bran is a psycho like me and I think that's kind of sweet. Now I don't have a mother again, but I'm fine. Nim doesn't have a mother either and look how happy he is! The whole Universe is his mother and right now he's having sex with her.

"Oooh, Bitch!" he moans. "Oooo, ooo, OOO!"

I look up and see my goddess Nicky coming across the lawn with a nice big breakfast tray for us and I signal for her to be quiet.

"Don't wake Nim, Nicky," I whisper. "He's having an orgy. You can watch if you like."

She bares all her teeth in a sexy smile and sets the tray down on ground and sits next to us trying to contain her amusement.

"Do you think he needs any help?" she teases.

"Nah. He's got complete control of this. But I need some help." I point to his arm around my throat and she gently pulls him off me.

She tears off a little piece of croissant and puts it in my mouth, then pours some coffee. Nim stops humming and kicking and sniffs. He smells it.

His eyes open halfway and he smiles decadently, purring and looking around not saying a word, looking at us in wonder.

"Howdya feel, Nim?" I really want to know.

"Still drunk," he laughs. "Coffee, please. Shoulda stuck to bourbon. Mmm, I slept out here last night? Did we—uh, I mean—shit, please don't tell me we three—again!?"

He looks horribly worried.

"No one touched you, baby," Nicky assures him. "Although you were all over Kama Dave this morning."

"Yeah," I laugh, "You were just fucking yourself and the Milky Way, Nim. You're fine."

"Oh. Alright then." He sits up and takes a cup of coffee from Nick. "Jesus," he moans feeling his face. His nose is crusty with blood. "What the fuck?"

"Oops, sorry. You did a couple face plants on the asphalt. And I punched you once. Hard to say which is responsible."

"Oh, thanks, brother. You punched me?"

"You hit me first. Sparring. You liked it, but I won. I'm getting awfully good."

Nicky takes a napkin, wets it with the dew from the lawn and starts cleaning his face, but he won't look at her. It's like he's afraid he'll fall into that deep green sea again and drown if he looks her in the eye.

"What's wrong, sweetheart?" she says softly. "Guilty?"

He shakes his head furiously. "That's a stupid emotion. Almost as useless as anger and jealousy."

"Then look at me, honey," she says. "Afraid?"

He looks up at her with a defiant sneer and laughs.

She tries again. "Confused?"

Now his frown fades and he just looks hopelessly lost and nods.

"Confused is good, S&M," she assures him. "If you think you've got everything under control, you're delusional. Trust me. I think confused is a pretty healthy emotion for you under the circumstances."

He doesn't talk. He just sips on the coffee thoughtfully and has a few bites of croissant.

"I heard every word you said yesterday, baby," she continues. "I understand what you're trying to do and I'm going to make every effort—I mean it—to be nicer to your wife. My sister.

"I have a sister I haven't seen in over ten years. I don't much like her and I only hear from her when she wants something. So I don't really know how to be a sister, but I'll try."

Nim looks at her with surprise.

"Is she half as beautiful as you, Nick?" he teases.

"Very beautiful, baby. And that got her into nothing but trouble. She got pregnant at 16 and a few more times, but she never kept any of them. Like I said, I haven't seen her in a long time. She'd be older than Mack now. She was a real train wreck."

"Thanks, Nick," he says. "I know Bran looks up to you. And I know Jack already loves his Aunt Nicky, so you might as well share him."

His face drains of color all of a sudden and I think he may be sick but he recovers.

"I mean—God, no! I mean share taking care of him."

"S&M, honey," she says. "I know I'm making you nervous. We're not sharing any more, not like we did. I didn't think it would upset you. You liked it before you knew I was your half-sister-in-law. And really, we're not even blood relatives, honey, it's only an ethical technicality.

"But I know it's bothering you now and I don't want to hurt you. I promise that Kamadev and I won't seduce you again. You'll have to beg us next time," she laughs.

"Yeah, Nim," I tease him. "You'll have to ask nicely 99 times."

"Thanks, guys," he grunts. "I did like it, very much. I'm grateful you shared with me, but it reminded me what I'm missing, what I need to work out. And I gladly accept your invitation to be your adopted boyfriend. We'll just keep it platonic. I don't need to sleep with you guys to know how much you love me. I won't ever forget."

He puts his left hand flat out on the lumpy sofa and looks in Nicky's emerald eyes. She puts her hand on his and then he looks at me. I put my hand on the stack and then Nim puts his right hand with the Om tattoo on top, making a sandwich of hands. Nick puts her right hand on top and I finish the tower of hands with mine.

"We're all adopting each other. Forever," he promises. "Brother, sister, friend, lover, slave, teacher, student, anything and everything, world without end. Done."

Nim gets up and stretches his hands to the sky then bends like a tree to one side and then the other. He pulls his knees into his chest one at a time and then hangs forward from his waist for a minute.

"Fine," he says. "Nicky, how do you feel about snakes?"

"Ew," she says. "I like them better dead. Snakeskin is very sexy."

"Thought so," he says. "I promised a kid I was going to go play with some snakes this morning. I guess you'll pass. Kamadev, have you got some time to play with snakes before work?"

†

BRANDY

It's my first night back in the pool house, but Sim never comes home. If I had known I would've slept on the cot in the nurses' room close to our little boy. Instead I sleep in the big bed alone. Even without him though, it's a huge relief to be back in our bedroom.

I have faith and hope. His favorite handcuffs are back on the shelf along with the spare key and I know, sooner or later, he'll miss them.

After all the sangria and food I was sleepy enough, but after listening to Nicky tell all the bedtime stories about Shiva, Parvati and Kamadev, I fall into deep dreams as soon as I lie down.

I dream I am Parvati, the beloved wife and favorite student of Shiva, his most cherished playmate. In the stories Nicky tells, Shiva loves to play dice with Parvati and cheats horribly, taking all her jewelry.

In turn, Parvati occasionally manages to win because the Universe loves justice, but Shiva refuses to accept defeat. It's not that Shiva really cares about the possessions and prizes, he just wants the game to go on perpetually.

The game, Nicky says, is a metaphor for the Universe. The play, the 'lila' of Shiva, represents the constant creation of Maya, the illusion of concrete reality, the dance of the world.

In my dream, I win every last bit of Sim's heart, every toy, every piece of property and clothing and even the dice themselves. Then I give everything back to him so we can play some more.

I'm deep into the dream when I hear voices in the bedroom. When I open my eyes, it's morning. Sim and Dave are smiling at me with a little breakfast tray.

"Sorry, beautiful girl," Sim growls. "I was useless last night. I hope you slept well."

He's got a little bit of a black eye and it looks nice on him. I smile and take the tray and smell the rich dark roast coffee with pleasure. Ah, breakfast in bed. Croissant, fresh fruit and cherry jam. Breakfast for one unfortunately.

“Gotta go, baby,” he apologizes. “Dave and I are going to take Jack down in the forest to play with Fang. I promised him. I’ll make sure he has a healthy breakfast. What do kids eat? I guess I’ll find out.”

“Anything with milk I think. You might hit it off with a protein shake. Banana, honey and peanut butter. Put some ice, cocoa powder and cinnamon in it and tell him it’s a milkshake.”

“Cool, beautiful,” he says. “I’ll see you soon. Doesn’t take all day to play with snakes. We have business you and I.”

He leaves, but he’s not gone. I feel him in the room like an echo. I get up and sit in the chair by the window and have my breakfast there, waiting and watching for a long time until I see them—Sim, Dave and Jack—crossing the lawn towards the forest, exploding with joy and laughter.

When they disappear, I go out on the deck to inspect the sorry struggling herb garden. I’ve only been gone a few days but the signs of neglect are already apparent. The thyme is completely dried on its sprigs, harvestable but dead. The tarragon leaves hang pitifully threatening suicide unless they get some attention.

I water the ones that can be saved, pull the thyme out of its pot and take it next door to present to the chef. Prince is serving breakfast to Nicky, Nat and Jain when I arrive, so I sit with them and have another cup of coffee.

I’m embarrassed. I don’t know how much they know about why I was missing for four days and I don’t want to explain. But the absence of questions tells me they probably know.

Nicky looks at me strangely and then smiles.

"Brandy, I apologize for being so harsh." Then she laughs. "My God, it sounds so funny to hear myself apologize. I don't do it much!

"I want to help you with Jack and if there is anything I can do to help with your husband, I know him pretty well."

Ah, shit, they know. They know he kicked me out of the house. They know it hasn't been working out well between us. I blush but thank her.

"I really don't know how you could help with Sim, Nicky, but thanks."

"Yeah," she says. "He's complicated. Good luck with that."

Nat waits until Prince leaves the room and puts a hand on my arm.

"I can help, Brandy. I don't know him as well as Nicky, but I know what's wrong."

"Really!" Nicky snorts.

"Yes, really," Nat says. "You're too close to Sim to see it, Nicky. And *your* beautiful boy is so talented you haven't had to deal with this. Sim is really confused about sex. It's that simple.

"So is Brandy. What she needs to learn is how to let him relax and enjoy it. A little bit of Tantra. He just doesn't know how to teach her."

"And you think you do?" Nicky challenges her.

"Nick. I taught Kamadev. Before you were interested in him. Before I was engaged. Sorry, Rick. I think my credentials speak for themselves. He's – Kamadev! He's a love god."

Jain looks pathetically at his plate and pushes his eggs around half-heartedly as she continues.

"Rick and I can give you a little guidance Brandy. It's not rocket science. If you've got an hour, we'd be happy to teach you some basics."

Jain drops his fork and looks at her with horror.

"Nat?" he mumbles. "I don't think so."

Nicky looks amused. "Mmm, you're going to give Brandy Tantra lessons? Interesting. I agree with you on one thing, Nat. He's a very confused boy right now. If you can help him, more power to you."

"So, Brandy," Nat turns to me, "has Sim tried to teach you any Tantra?"

"Yes. He taught me my chakras. And I—uh," I don't know if I should say this in front of Nicky but I'm desperate for help.

"Sim gave up on me, Nat, but Dave gave me some advice that worked. 'Pay attention to the fire at the beginning in order to avoid the embers at the end.' And Sim said that was a good start."

"Dave is teaching you?" Nicky hisses.

I just nod with my eyes averted submissively.

"That's good advice," Nat ignores her. "So we're going to work on kindling the fire and keeping it from burning too hot and comsuming everything.

"Sim taught you *your* chakras, but I'm going to teach you *his* chakras—the ones you don't have."

"Oooo fuck," Rick moans.

"What do you mean, Nat?" Nicky wonders.

"The lingam chakras, Nicky. A man's sex."

"I don't know about that," she complains. "Why don't I know about that?"

"You haven't needed to know, Nicky," Nat continues. "Your boy doesn't need relaxing. He hasn't got an ounce of negative conditioning. You don't need to learn this."

"Oh, but I want to! I have my fair share of challenges with Dave. I want to know everything about making him happy."

Nat shrugs and smiles at Jain who is shaking his head in disbelief.

†

## JAIN

Now, I'm not shy. I'm a doctor. But a Tantric sex lesson is intimate and I'm not at all comfortable with teaching these beautiful women how it works.

"Oh, come on, Doc!" Nicky begs. "It's not like we haven't seen it before. I mean – not you, but you know. I'm married."

"Rick," Nat explains, "this is absolutely not sexual, it's clinical, therapeutic. You were Brandy's mentor for nursing school. You're a great teacher.

"And you weren't at all shy about cutting me open and taking a look at my internal organs! Think of this as surgery—except no one is going to cut you."

She laughs at the painful look on my face.

"Do you want to put your old buddy Sim out of his misery or not? Give us an hour of your time. You're just going to be our surrogate dummy."

She knows I can't say no. I'm not happy but I'll do it. Prince comes back in the room and clears the plates and for a hot second, I wonder if they could use him instead.

Other than the fact that he's not an adult, he's a virgin, and he's painfully erotophobic—okay maybe it wouldn't work.

"Brandy, are you comfortable with working on Rick – um, Dr. Jain?"

She nods seriously. "He's my teacher. I trust him."

"How about you, Nicky?"

"Oooh, yeah," she leers. "More than comfortable."

"Nicky, it's supposed to be non-sexual," she says. "Do you have any physical attraction?"

"Absolutely. Look at him, Nat. He's beyond beautiful. If my husband is made out of sugar, yours is made out of Kobe beef. But I can contain myself."

She winks at me. My heart sinks all the way beyond my stomach but I'm amused. I don't get to eat Kobe beef very often in the Fire House but it's considered the most exclusive beef in the world.

The cattle are pampered like spoiled children, massaged daily and plied with sake and beer. The theory is that a relaxed mellow cow makes better beef. Maybe a relaxed mellow man makes better love.

Nat has mercy on me and lets me go in the lab ahead of them to undress and get on the massage table. I feel eerily like a patient left alone to don a hospital gown but all I've got is a sheet.

A few minutes later, the ladies come in and Nat puts a little yoga pillow over my eyes.

"Just relax and keep your eyes closed, but tell us if anything is uncomfortable or painful or nice. Feedback is important."

Strangely enough, I find myself relaxing deeply, easily. I know this. I know it doesn't go anywhere; it's just pleasant. My mind drifts gently as I hear her explaining the anatomy of my sexual apparatus and the energetic workings of the penile chakras.

It's almost like a concentrated yoga nidra as she names my bits and pieces. My mind wanders through my physical inventory and begins to tune itself out. By the time she actually lays one of her hands on my heart and the other hand on top of the sheet on my sex organs, I'm already miles away.

All the feedback they get from me is "Ah, oo, oh and mmm." I turn into an Om synthesizer. Even when the hands go under the sheet and all over the place I don't mind. I can't really tell who's touching me.

Then all of a sudden I'm yanked back into the room with a jolt.

"Jesus, Nicky!" I moan. "Turn the heat down for God's sake!"

"How do you know it's me?" she asks innocently? "What am I doing wrong?"

"It's supposed to be easy, honey," I instruct her. "Not like that!"

Brandy and Nat massage like therapists but Nicky massages like a sex freak. Shit!

"Sorry," she says. "It looks like it's built to be treated like that. Feels like it too."

†

## JACK

I'm lost when I wake up but then I see I'm in my own new room in a sweet little bed. The very complicated puzzle is on the floor for me to play with.

I'm all alone but that's okay. My old mother left me alone a lot. I get down on the floor and watch the puzzle. It looks too hard for me but I like seeing the picture coming out of it, a beautiful pond with flowers floating on it like little boats and trees dipping into the water.

I look all around the picture for snakes or birds but I can't even find a fish.

After a while, I put on my new jeans and Point Guard shirt and tip toe down the stairs. My Uncle Dr. Mack is sitting in his office. He smiles and invites me to sit on the big leather sofa, so big my feet can't touch the ground.

I start calming myself with the little finger signs: thumb and first finger together, the thumb and second finger, third finger, little baby finger.

Uncle Mac laughs, “Where did you learn that, Jack?”

“From my father.”

“Good for him. Do you know what they mean?” he asks.

“I know this one, wisdom,” I show him the okay sign. “A circle and three fingers counting my blessings. Dad says the rest come later.”

“Let me tell you the others then. I taught them to your father. The thumb and second finger is for patience and being happy with things just the way they are.

“The thumb and third finger is for health and energy. And with the little finger it helps seeing and saying things clearly.”

I test the fingers and count: wise, happy, healthy, clear. I smile at him with thanks.

“Good age to learn, don’t you think?” I hear my father say and look up to see him with Uncle Kama Dave in the doorway.

Dad has a black eye and he looks very happy. Dad and Uncle Dave both have scruffy faces like they forgot to shave. I wonder if he forgot his promise.

“Mack, we’re going to play with the creatures in the forest this morning,” he laughs. “I’ll just fix him a milkshake first.”

Oh, YES! He remembered. No one remembers promises! I squirm with happiness and hold my thumb and second finger together up to him and he smiles with approval and goes out to the kitchen.

Uncle Dave sits down beside me. He never stops smiling. My father looks very serious sometimes because he is in charge of everything but Uncle Kama Dave is just wildly happy like a free animal.

In a few minutes, Dad comes back with big milkshakes for everyone, chocolate banana peanut flavored. Uncle Mack is surprised but he tastes it and likes it.

Uncle Dave says, “We already had breakfast, Nim.”

“Yeah, but you’re a growing boy, little brother,” Dad laughs. “You can’t get bigger muscles eating croissants and jam.”

Dad flexes his arms and they pop up like mountains. We drink the shakes up and I tell my Uncle Mack about Fang, the giant king snake. As I tell it, Fang gets even bigger, now as long as my father.

Uncle holds his thumb and little finger together and smiles at me. Seeing things and saying things clearly. Oh. I understand and correct myself.

“Not really as big as Dad,” I apologize, “but maybe it will grow up, too.”

“Let’s go, little scrap,” Dad says. “Fang only plays in the morning. When the sun gets a little warmer, it’s lunch time and nap time for both of you!”

Dad and Uncle Dave take my hands and we go outside into the beautiful mountain top that looks like heaven with a pool and a gym. Then down the trail, much further than I’ve ever been but still I don’t see Fang.

“Sit,” Dad instructs. “If you wait long enough, everything will come around.”

We sit and sit and sit. Nobody talks. Dad closes his eyes and puts his fingers together with the sign of patience and happiness. Uncle Kama Dave just grins.

I see a little lizard sitting on a rock near us doing little lizard pushups. It's very funny to watch the tiny little creature. I wonder if he is just squirming by pushing up and down or if he's really trying to make some little muscles.

"Lizard lunch," Uncle Dave laughs. "That's what your big snake likes to eat for lunch."

"Oh, no!" I moan. "I don't want him eaten! He's trying so hard to be stronger!"

"Well, not that one then," he explains. "He's working out so hard, he'll be fast enough to get away. Fang will eat the slackers, the lazy lizards."

Suddenly the little lizard pops up and runs. I see my beautiful red snake crawl onto my father's bended knee and lift its head to look at me. Dad doesn't even open his eyes, but he puts a hand down to pet Fang gently.

I want to cry with happiness. I thought that Fang was the most beautiful thing I've ever seen but my father is a million times cooler. Even with a scruffy face and black eye, he shines with the sunlight washing all over him and the pretty snake on his lap. The snake has gotten very, very small now. It can never be as big as my father no matter how many slacker lizards it eats.

†

SEAN

Was that too good to be real? I wonder. I dropped Jack off at the Mack house like he was as expected as a pizza delivery. I would worry except I remember dropping Dave off with three felonies, dropping Nicky off drunk with a broken nose and seven toes and—I didn't actually drop the little heroin dealer Prince off, but now he's a brilliant chef. Sim seems to absorb trouble like a sponge.

I decide to go back up there today anyway. Not that I don't trust Sim, I just love him and want to say hi. I swing by Nicky's old cottage on the way up, check in with her landlord in the big house, collect her mail and send her regards.

Her place has been vacant since I hauled her up from the parking lot behind the Nest bar but the rent has been paid. Sim's been paying her bills since day one when he first met her. I always wondered why he didn't just move her into his beach house, but I figured it was a special relationship between them, something different.

When I get to Sunrise, I stop in to see Mack first. "It's crazy, Sean," he says. "Steven's a natural born father. Maybe not a great husband, but I think he's a very gifted father."

Mack calls the Fire House and asks Prince to serve lunch by the pool. When we go out on the lawn Nicky, Brandy, Nat and Jain are already lounging about in the sunshine. Jain is getting the royal massage treatment from his beautiful wife.

I give the little stack of mail to Nicky and she flicks through it quickly. She never gets a bill. She's got that covered, or rather Sim has. It's all junk except one personal letter and she opens it with a frown. She reads it and throws it on the ground, then picks it up again and reads it once more.

"Bitch!" she swears. "Always and forever a useless bitch."

This time she crumples it up in her hands and rolls it into a little ball. She throws it on the ground again and stares at it like she could incinerate it with her eyes.

"Hey, Nicky," I say. "Sorry to bring bad news. I'm just a courier. Everything looks good at your place."

"Sean," she sighs, "everything is good. Nothing that ever comes from her is good, so it's not really news."

She leans down and picks up the paper ball and throws it at me with a serious stare.

"See for yourself."

I don't want to mess around with her personal affairs, but it's an invitation as a friend. Maybe I can help. I smooth the letter out and read.

*My Dearest Sister,*

*I came by to see you but the landlord says you've been away. Where are you? I am desperately in need of money. I know you have a rich boyfriend who pays all your bills. Can't you help your poor sister with a little $$? I'll be around town for a while. I finally found the prick who ruined my life and once I get him to pay, I'll be gone. But until then I need some money. You owe your dear sister. OXO Diana*

"My Dearest Sister, shit!" she hisses. "My only sister and I never hear from her unless she needs money. Burn that, Sean honey."

I start to put a match to it but Mack stops me.

"Can I help her, Nicky?" he says. "If she needs money, we've got it. I don't mind. Let me take a look at it."

Nick doesn't flinch so I hand Mack the letter. As if the power shuts down in the middle of dinner, Mack groans and smacks the letter down.

"Diana. Oh, God," he moans. "Diana D? Diana Dixon?"

And even though Prince is bringing out a tray of sandwiches and lemonade, Mack gets to his feet and reaches out for Nicky's hand.

"Nicky, honey. We need to have a word in private. It won't take long, but it might ruin your appetite."

"Sorry, Mack," she hisses. "I learned my lesson a long time ago. I'm not letting that bitch ruin my life, my day or even my lunch. It's just not that important to me."

Prince puts the sandwiches down and the conversation quickly turns to saffron egg salad with tarragon and thyme. Diana D. dissolves back into obscurity but Mack folds the letter up carefully and puts it in his pocket with a frown.

†

## BRANDY

My heart skips when I see them walking across the lawn. Dave and Jack are laughing uproariously; Sim is walking seriously and purposefully like a stripper. Oh my beautiful boys, honing in on the sandwiches like guided missiles.

The younger two grab sandwiches with both hands, but Sim waits, knowing Prince will keep the food coming as long as it takes.

He walks around behind Nicky's chair and puts his hands on her shoulders, squeezing them hard and massaging the anger and tension right out of her. I see her face soften with relief and her eyelids close. But when I look up at Sim, his hands are on her but his eyes are all over me, piercing, teasing.

My God, he's playing with me. When he catches my eye his mouth turns up on the left edge in a snarl and he shows me his pretty, sharp canine tooth. Then he licks his lips slowly, methodically, and bares all his teeth in a smile calculated to blind any living female within his range.

I feel his hands vicariously on me through her and I nearly moan with pleasure. I almost forget the lesson Nat just gave us about lowering the heat of passion to a slow simmer. His desire is igniting my spine and melting my sinews.

Holy honey, it takes all I've got to rein in my resolve and concentrate.

'Do you want to tend the fire or do you just want to burn up all the wood?' he asked me two days ago. I want the fire to burn forever. I can do this. The Tantrika didn't let me put my hands on her beautiful husband for nothing.

I've completely lost my appetite for egg salad. I compose myself and get to my feet. Tearing my eyes off him, I walk away back to the pool house. I don't even have to turn around to know he's following me home. I can feel his eyes burning my back like the lash of a whip.

†

## S&M

Once we're inside I throw myself down on the big bed. I'm ready to tear her world apart.

"What am I going to do with you, little girl?" I tease hooking my thumbs under the waistband of my leather pants. I can turn her to stone with insinuation alone.

But she pulls herself up tall and folds her hands together in front of her heart.

"No, Sim," she insists. "What am I going to do with *you*? I've been studying with Nat. I think you'll like it."

Oh. My curiosity is piqued. What has she got for me this time?

"Mmm," I snort. "It better have nothing to do with handcuffs or hypodermic needles, little nurse, because technically you are still on probation. It's barely been a week since you attacked me, baby."

"Trust me," she purrs. "Come outside." Famous last words but I get up and follow her out through the kitchen to the yoga deck. She spreads a sheet on the massage table.

"No sex right now. Just strip, Sim."

I leer at her as I untie my belt and pull the pants off but she averts her eyes. I wonder what kind of game she's playing. She's missing the best show on Earth and I'm slightly offended that she isn't watching me, but I lie down on the table and exhale.

When she covers me, I realize it's actually a relief that the show is over and my performance is apparently cancelled. I've never for one moment relaxed with her: it's always been a full-on show, a spectacular over-the-top sexual extravaganza. Even simply gazing into her soul was an orchestrated Tantric ritual. I close my eyes and listen to the wind in the trees and feel her hands on me, one on my forehead, one on my heart.

"Just relax, Sim," she whispers. "No expectations; nowhere to go, nothing to do. Just let me hold you. Trust me."

She moves her right hand down to my groin and the left hand to my heart and she just holds them there motionless. I can feel the connection between my heart chakra and my pelvic chakra and my energy flares between her hands on a slow simmer.

I can come just like this but I wait and relax, counting my breaths from 99 backwards. Around 74, she moves her right hand to my cock. Still.

Motionless. How the hell can she feel me like that and not do anything? What is Nat teaching her?

How can my little nymphomaniac wife resist taking a big bite out of me? I'm amazed by her control and restraint. Now both her hands go down on me, softly massaging all my bits and pieces, brushing away the tension, easing my lust.

It's sweet. Somehow she's managed to take all the urgency out of her caress. Oh, sweet milk and honey, she's getting into the transcendental aspect. She's finally diving down into the cake.

I'm counting to 59 backwards. I'm counting to 96 upside down. I'm floating on top of numbers and breathing softer and silkier and deeper.

I don't drop down deep like I do with yoga nidra. Instead I feel myself rising up to the rafters and looking down at my body from above. Damn, it's a beautiful looking corpse in spite of the gunshot scars!

I look like a dead man, a very beautiful dead man. She pets me and strokes me with such devoted attention she doesn't even realize that I'm gone.

†

## SHIVA

Sita is lying on the ground right where I set her down. She's been dead for a very long time but I can't bear to part with her body. I lift her over my shoulder again and continue carrying her but one of her arms drops off. When I bend down to pick it up, a foot falls off as well.

It makes me furious that I can't keep her in one piece! I walk for days, at last setting her down under a sacred ashoka tree and she loses a whole leg. I haven't got enough hands to carry all her pieces now so I just howl with misery and sit next to her.

I will never get up again. The whole Universe can go to hell. I'm no longer concerned with it. Eternity passes as I sit in penance, mourning her loss. The Universe unravels just as her body has.

Kamadev sits at my feet and begs me to get back up and turn the wheel of the world but I spit at him. He goes away and comes back with another wife for me and begs me to stop crying.

She is just another woman who means nothing to me. I can't teach her what she needs to know because my heart has fallen apart like the Universe.

Kamadev plucks flowers from the ashoka tree, scoops lotus blossoms from the water and pulls sprigs of jasmine from his hair. He ties them all together to his bow and shoots me. I want to die so I'm grateful when the arrow pierces my heart, but instead of death he's injected me with powerful lust.

I feel my pulse racing and my blood burning. My eyes are fixed now on this new woman, more intoxicating than opium perfumes.

"Damn you, Kamadev!" I roar before I pounce upon my new wife. I focus my rage like a laser through my third eye and burn the boy alive, toasted to a crisp, incinerated to cold ashes by the heat of my passion.

Then I begin to take my new wife in every position possible and start teaching her everything that she needs to know. It will take a very long time.

†

## DJ

He's growing on me. I cried the first time I saw him because I wanted Nim for myself, but now it's even better with two new brothers, a new sister and best of all this little scrap of Nim's, my nephew.

Jack looks like me, like the little me before I ran away from my evil parents. How could they be so mean when I was little like that, just wanting to play and be protected?

I hate to think about my fake parents. My first mother was so beautiful like Nicky but I can hardly remember her. When I was just little she gave me to the bad ones. She was very mad at me and threw me away.

I thought Nim would throw me away when he got Jack, but now we play more. And now he loves Brandy again. I saw his eyes sparkle and shine on her when he was rubbing Nicky's shoulders. He has plenty of love for all of us now and I don't think he will throw any of us away.

When Nim follows Brandy home, I have plenty of good choices. I can play some more with Jack or have a nice massage with Nat or work in the lab. But maybe I should have a nap with Nicky.

Sean shakes my hand and laughs, "I meant to check in with Sim but he seems too busy. Are you doing okay, Dave? No problems with your rehab?"

"I'm stunning, Sean!" I tell him. "I've got a new job working in the lab! No drugs, just nice plant medicines. Nat is teaching me how to be a—uh…" I look to her for help.

"A very talented mad scientist, Sean," she teases. "He's very astute."

"And! I'm going to be on the Board when I'm done with probation!"

"For real?" Sean turns to Mack. "You're making him a partner?"

"For real," Mack smiles. "We're keeping him, Sean."

"Man, that's good news, Dave," he says. "You *are* stunning, buddy. I'm blown away."

"Hmm," Mack adds. "No junkies, no blood shed, no intensive care patients at the moment. What the hell are we going to do with ourselves?"

"I could always bring you some more trouble, Mack," he teases. "We've got plenty of it downtown. Steven's old buddy Billy Lee is going right off the deep end right now."

"Not today, thanks," Mack says.

"Jack needs a nap," I suggest.

I make a face at Nicky like I'm a poor lonely lost boy and she nods her head at me with a luscious smile. Maybe there will be no nap at all. Maybe I'll just invent some new games to play with her.

Nicky gets up and wraps her arms around my shoulders and whispers in my ear. It tickles me.

Jack groans, "I think you're in trouble, Uncle Dave."

"I hope so, little scrap." I wink at him. "Deep dark trouble."

†

## NAT

I'm just helping Prince clean up in the kitchen when the phone rings. Brandy—the calmest coolest nurse I've ever met—is frantic.

"Nat, he's dead!" she moans. "He quit breathing! Oh, God, help me. Please, please."

"I'm coming," I hang up on her and grab Rick on the way over. If Sim's dead, a doctor won't help much but I wouldn't mind a second opinion.

Brandy meets us at the door and points out back. Sim is laid out like a corpse on the massage table with a sheet covering him. He's not breathing but he's got a smile as big as Texas on his lips.

Rick checks his pulse.

"Mmm, he's not dead. But his pulse is barely 40," he says. "What happened?"

"Just what we did," she moans. "What Nat taught us. Uh—Tantric massage. He just stopped breathing."

Rick checks his pupils. They're dilated to black pools with only the slightest blue rim around the edges. There's no discernable breath.

"Shit, I don't know," he swears. "I know it made me kind of floaty but—he looks like he's on drugs. It's like a trance. I don't think that's a medical diagnosis though."

"He's fine," I assure them. "It's a good diagnosis, Doctor. Maybe you just got floaty, but this is Sim here. Mr. Transcendental.

"You did a good job, Brandy. He's not dead but he's definitely crossed over to the other side—probably taking care of some celestial business. We can stay with you if you like, but all you really need to do is wait for him to come back down."

"He's fine?" she sobs. "Are you sure?"

"Yogis stop breathing. On a good day if he's just hanging out, he's probably taking 3 or 4 breaths a minute. That's normal. He's just breathing so slow you don't notice.

"You're going to like it when he comes back. You've just recharged his Tantric batteries and kick started his kundalini. We'll keep an eye on Jack for you. You're going to have your hands full tonight."

†

## MACK

Sunny is curled up on the big leather couch in my office next to Jack. He's been up since dawn and I can see his eyes drooping towards a nap. She pets his hair and offers to tuck him in.

"Your father is resting for a while with your mother," she says.

"Yeah. Sex. I know," he rolls his eyes.

"Oh?" I wonder. "What's a nine year old boy know about sex?"

"Seen it," he sighs with boredom. "Seen it a lot. Looks like a lot of trouble."

"Uh." I'm a bit shocked. "Your mother?"

"Yep. She wasn't shy. Lots of boyfriends. Lots and lots of trouble. Sex and drugs and no fucking rock'n roll."

Sunny's mouth drops and she looks at me for support but I'm just as disturbed.

"What? What?" he says. "I didn't say it at the table!"

"Nap time, Jack," I say. "Sunny will tuck you in."

Jack holds his fingers up to me in the Gyan mudra of wisdom: 'okay'. Whatever crappy upbringing the kid had, he has Steven's blood and genes. He has distance. He has impervious distance.

While Sunny takes him upstairs, I brood over the letter. I need to talk to someone but I don't know who. Everything appears to be falling into place, every happily ever after dream is settling on the top of the mountain, but there are things I don't want to know.

Sim is in love with his wife again. Jack is safe with us. And Kama Dave—ah, shit. My little brother is tearing my heart open, the crazy beautiful boy. I thought we put his plight to rest. We've kept him out of prison and set him up financially. He's married to the girl of his dreams and—now I think—she could become his nightmare.

"Sunshine," I sigh as Sunny comes back into the office. "I need to talk to someone. You're probably the only one up here who isn't involved.

"Can you help me with this, honey?"

I hand her the letter and let her drink it in. It isn't much on it's own, just a whining begging relative, apparently one who's not much liked by her dear sister.

"That one's from Nicky's sister," I tell her. "And this one I ignored because it sucks and it's misappropriated. It's addressed to me but most likely intended for my deceased father. Ah, it truly sucks, Sunny."

I hand her a letter forwarded from the hospital a few weeks ago in identical handwriting.

*Dr. David Mack,*

*At last I've tracked you down you bastard. I should have sent you to prison after all. You promised to support me and your son, you liar! And then you just cut us off after 6 years. Well fuck you! I gave him away because I couldn't stand to be reminded of you!*

*It's too late to press charges but I can make your life hell if you don't pay. I can ruin you. It was statutory rape after all. I was only 16 and you predator bastard were 33 with a wife and kids. You can't get away with this. Make it right or burn in hell.*

*Diana D.*

"Mack? What??" she says confused. It's too complicated to wrap her mind around it.

"When I got this letter, I knew it wasn't for me. But I thought of—Dad. We have the same name. Hell, Dave is named after him, too. I did the math and figured Dave was his son. He didn't cut her off; he fucking died. And I thought I made everything right by making Dave a partner and taking care of him.

"But now—Jesus! This new letter to Nicky! If Diana is Nicky's sister and also Dave's mother, it's disturbing. He's married to his aunt. Of course there's no proof. Dad might have had a hundred kids like Steven. Maybe she's not his mother but—damn, Sunny. I'm confused."

"Ooh shit," she says absorbing it all. "Not good. Not even legal."

"Yeah," I groan. "That's what I thought. It could send Kama Dave to a mental hospital if he finds out he's not married. Little Jack got it right. Sex is a lot of trouble."

## Part Three: BLOOD AND MERCY

**"To touch is to heal,**
**to hurt is to steal**
**If you want to kiss the sky,**
**better learn how to kneel**
**On your knees, boy!"**
**~ U2**

# Part Three: Blood and Mercy

†

## PRINCE ALBERT

I haven't seen Cat in a week. I told her I'm busy and of course I am with all the shopping, planning, cooking, serving and cleanup for 10 people. She can text me. It's a whole lot safer. We can joke and flirt and talk but she can't touch me.

I think that's a hell of a lot better than dating. After Dr. Jain explained all the complications, rules and provisions for safe sex, including jail since she's only seventeen, I think texting is very smart.

The day before yesterday the police brought one of S&M's kids over to live with us! Back when he was trying to talk to me about sex he said he has a hundred of them! What would happen if they all showed up for dinner? How would we ever feed them?

I told Cat she can text me after dinner between 8 and 9 and maybe come over once in a while, but no dates. The trouble is, even though she's not a consenting adult, she's extremely consensual.

Kama Dave knocks on my door after lunch and asks if he can borrow my little portable speakers and I-pod for his nap. Why the hell does he need music for a nap? But he gives me fifty bucks to borrow it for a couple hours.

He has no clue how much money is worth, but he's got a job now and he's made some off his fake casino bank so he's got the green stuff. I would have let him borrow it for $5, but I take the Ulysses S. Grant greenback off him anyway. The guy has to learn about money one of these days.

I show him how to work it and he asks me to cue it up to Def Leppard. 'Pour Some Sugar on Me.' That's not exactly nap material but then that's why we call him Psycho Dave.

Now everybody seems to be napping but me. Dr. and Mrs. Jain have disappeared, Dr. Mack and Sunny took Jack home, Sean left, and S&M went home with his wife.

I could go shopping or I could—hmm, maybe she misses me. I try a little text.

*How is the Cat girl?*

She doesn't answer so I start making a shopping list. Tonight it's going to be lamb enchiladas. S&M loves them. Spanish rice and black beans. No sangria for them tonight, they get too crazy on that.

Instead I'm going to serve wine spritzers which is just watered down wine with fruit garnish. They all need to take it easy and they won't know the difference.

The phone buzzes so I look.

*The Cat girl is lonely!!! What's for dinner, Chef Prince?*

Well, she's not shy, inviting herself for dinner, but she can't come over when everyone is taking a nap because it could get dangerous by myself.

*Sorry my boss is having a private adult party. Maybe tomorrow.*

I lie, but it's pretty convenient. Adults only. She'll be curious about what's going on. She texts back right away.

*I want to go to S&M's private adult party! Waaah!*

*Behave!* I text back. She's too young for me, I think; but more than anything, I don't want to share him with her.

I turn the phone off and go look in the kitchen to see if I've got the goods for dinner. I've got lamb shanks and the works so I get down to cooking. Shanks are too easy. Once they're prepped they just go in the oven until they fall off the bone while the chef kicks his heels up.

While I'm prepping, I can hear Def Leppard pounding over and over again upstairs on repeat. *'I'm hot. Sticky sweet from my head to my feet...you got the peaches, I got the cream'*

It sounds like a dessert recipe but I don't think that's what Dave is cooking up. I decide to make a peach cobbler with whipped cream for dessert as a snide joke to see if he gets it.

But man he's already getting it. As the song fades out, I hear her screaming. It sounds complicated. I've never heard such happy screaming before. And then the song starts all over again.

†

## S&M

Dusk or dawn, I couldn't say which it is. It's that magic dirty hour between light and darkness when everything just melts. She's sitting on the futon cross-legged watching out for me, watching over me, watching someone else she thinks is me.

I'm the Nataraj turning the world. I've seen her dead and falling to pieces. I've seen her out of control and ravenous and now I'm just watching someone else watching me. Who the fuck is she? Someone new I think. A new wife for me. Pretty soft brown eyes and golden hair and skin as deep and dark as carmel crème.

"Ah, Sim," she sighs. "Are you all right, baby? I was worried."

"Why don't you see for yourself?" I tease her. I don't really think I know her. "*Am* I all right?"

I get off the table and stand in front of her but she's not scared. She should be. Who am I? I was dead but now I'm burning up. I lie down on the futon and take her wrists and then I take her mouth and then everything. Slowly. World without end.

She likes it very much. I can't really take anything from her because she's just giving it up to me so freely. She matches me breath for breath, move for move. This is a damn good wife this time. I hope she doesn't fall apart on me.

I bite her lip and she bites me back, everything perfectly orchestrated on queue. I squeeze all of the air out of her lungs and she inhales me. She fits me perfectly like a second skin.

Her heartbeat is synchronized to mine, slowly, very slowly pumping in time to my rhythm like a drum. The Universe is turned on again.

†

## BRANDY

He was out for nearly six hours. When he wakes he looks like another man, a crazy ravenous man. His eyes are half-closed and dreamy like a junkie and right away I'm reminded of the way DJ looked after he became Kamadev. Experienced. Not just stoned, but beautiful.

Sim looks intoxicated and sedated—like he looked when I drugged him with lorezepam—alarmingly compliant and willing.

It worries me but when I ask how he is, he says to see for myself. And then he lies down next to me and starts putting out like he's never done before. Without his crazy mantras and rules, without control or instructions, without games or toys, he just plain lights the fire and stokes it steadily.

He's turning into the sexual legend I've always suspected him capable of being. Love has nothing to do with it. He's always been a loving man, but now he's unleashed his inhibitions, without restraint and even without lust. It's just pure surrender and submission to femininity.

"Mother!" he moans. "Am I all right?"

"You're perfect, baby," I assure him. "Divine perfection."

†

## MACK

Tonight's dinner is a bit more sedate. Steven doesn't show up but I take that as a good omen since he's with his wife. Kama Dave comes down to the dinner table dressed in more clothing than I've even seen on him, accessorized to the teeth with everything a boy could possibly wear except shoes and a shirt.

He's got his leathers and silks and gloves and half of her jewelry and flowers and—his finest accessory—his sultry playmate on his arm. His wife or his aunt? Legally she can't be both. Not in *this* state. I really don't want to know the details.

I pull out a chair for him at the head of the table. He looks surprised, but his eyes sparkle with joy as he surveys the motley crew around the table.

"Where's Nim?" he wonders.

"Honeymoon," I say. "Can you take his place tonight as the honorary head of the Fire House?"

"Absolutely. Sure," he smiles scrutinizing the pack.

"Straighten up, Jack," he commands. "Do you want more wine, Nat? Prince, can you get more salad for the south end of the table?"

Kama Dave starts barking out orders as if he's assumed Steven's role controlling the Universe. His mannerisms, his facial expression and his tone all change. I have to look twice to remind myself it's still Dave.

It reminds me of something Steven once told me: *There is no better plan for a person who needs supervision than to give them someone else to supervise. All the guardian angels in the cosmos are probably celestial derelicts watching over errant humans. Minding someone else's business can keep you out of the deep end of trouble.*

Now I think I understand why Steven tries so hard to keep the whole Universe organized and running smoothly. It's his personal plan to save himself.

At the end of the meal, Prince clears away the dishes and brings out a big tray of peach cobbler and a bowl of whipping cream, presenting the dessert in front of Dave.

Dave stares at it for a minute and then starts howling with laughter. He peels his gloves off slowly like a stripper, leering at his playmate/wife/auntie.

He nearly puts his nose into the bowl of cream and breathes it deeply and slowly.

"Well done, Chef," he purrs. "You've put rosewater and saffron in the cream. Brilliant aphrodisiacs."

Then he scoops up a serving of the rich whipping cream with his bare hand and holds it out to Nicky. She snarls at him wickedly and slowly licks his hand clean.

"Jesus!" Prince protests. "Not at the table!"

"You started it, Prince Albert," Dave snorts. "How much do you want for the little music player?"

"Uh—how about $750?" Prince tries. I happen to know he bought it with his Sunrise online account for about a hundred bucks.

"Cool," Dave laughs. "$700 then. I already gave you fifty. She likes it very much with the music. You should probably go whip up another batch of cream for the rest of the table."

†

## DJ

Nim doesn't want anything to do with me this morning, but I keep pounding on the pool house door until he finally opens it—naked.

"What, what, WHAT the fuck?" he snarls. "What can't wait for me to finish up?"

"It's never finished, Nim," I remind him. "You don't have to do it all at once. You taught me that."

"Yeah? Well I'm just getting started. It took me seven years to sort this shit out. I think I've got it figured out. Fuck off, little brother."

I don't argue with him. I know that never works. I just make a face at him like I'm a poor lost boy all alone. I've got a patent pending on that look.

He stares at me and cools off a little.

"Geez, Kamadev, look at you. It's only 6am and you're dressed like a whore."

"Nah, like a stripper! I got my music going now and everything, Nim. You were so right. It's making her scream."

"Hmmpf," he nods. "Thought so. Nicky's easy. I'll bet she likes that even better than whipping you to see if you love her. As long as she's getting 110% of your attention, she's easy."

"Look, man," I say in my best imitation of Nim controlling the Universe, "I'm terribly busy myself today but I'm taking a break so we can play with Jack before I have to go back—to work. Let's go."

He rolls his eyes but he puts on his sweat pants, "Don't go anywhere, woman," he yells over his shoulder.

Man, Nim looks terrible today, worse than he looked hung over, but I don't tell him that. He looks disorganized and totally disintegrated. On the way over to Mack's house, I give him a little bottle of 'Rx Jack' to sniff so he can calm down.

I hope he's not getting into straight sex now because that can kill a man—or at least knock the wind out of him. I don't want to lose my teacher.

Nim sits with Dr. Mack while I fix our shakes for breakfast. We're not supposed to drink the oils, but Nat made some tinctures, which are okay. She gave me a little bottle of tulsi.

"Trust me," she said with a wink, "Tulsi has a lot of amazing properties but it's especially nice for emotional scars. For you-know-who."

Oh. I-know-exactly-who is hurting himself with remorse. Why not? I put a lot of it in the shake and switch out the peanut butter for tahini. And then hell, I put a few drops of the lavender in too. It's supposed to balance strength and femininity.

You-know-who can stand a little more balance in that department. Then I add in a lot of fresh cherries. Nat says there's some inflammatory compound in cherries that helps with pain and Nim is my new science project now.

I give the shakes to everyone and grin while I drink mine. I can't wait to see what it does to us. I'm getting calmer and stronger and mellower and more receptive just thinking about it.

After breakfast, I lead the way down to the grove. It's just me, Jack and Nim. "Down to the pond?" I suggest.

"Nah, nah, naught," he commands. "The little scrap doesn't know how to swim yet. This is fine. This is far enough."

"A pond? A pond? Like the picture puzzle?" Jack nearly squirms out of his skin.

"NO!" Nim glares around at the Universe like he might kill every bit of it.

He sits down hard on the forest floor and pulls his legs beneath him.

"Dad? Baby?" Jack moans. "I really want a pond. Ooooh!"

"Ah, shit," Nim swears. "I give up. Kamadev, brother, I fucking quit. It's your game, baby. Lead the way."

We haven't been down to the pond since the day after Nicky and I loved him. I'll never forget. She won't. He won't. But damn. Once was enough. I wink at him and he stops breathing for a minute. He looks like he's going to punch me, but then he softens up and grins. The lavender must be working.

When we get to the water, Jack gasps in delight. He prowls all around it's edges with so much nervous excitement Nim can't contain his own joy anymore. Every little insect on the surface makes the kid squeal. He's hopelessly in love.

"Go on, strip, you little scrap," Nim instructs him. "It's not deep enough to drown you."

Jack gapes in disbelief but he pulls his little shirt off while watching his father step out of his sweat pants and plunge in among the water lilies. Nim floats his feet above the water and smiles in amusement as Jack strips off his jeans and tip toes into the cool water.

"Look at you, Jack. You don't even know who you are," Nim laughs. "You don't know where Jack ends and where the world begins. It's like there's no boundary, no separation at all."

"Good one, Nim," I laugh. "You're catching on."

His eyes go dark and deep for a minute as if he's looking inside his own head and then he gives me a piercing look.

"You didn't know who the fuck you were either did you, Kamadev? You didn't have a clue. That's how you disappeared so easily wasn't it?"

I nod and laugh at him. That's the secret to sex. I know how to disappear.

"That's why you love everybody so much, isn't it?" he continues. "You don't know where Kama Dave ends and where the world begins. There's no difference to you."

Now he gets a serious wink from me. I mean it. I love him. He's getting pretty damn smart for an older guy. He shakes his head in disbelief.

"I was worried sick about disappearing. I was making sex too complicated because I was disappearing in it. I was just trying so hard to keep it under control. Fuck it. Fuck everything."

"You've got it, Nim," I assure him. "You're supposed to get lost. That's the point. You taught me that. Tat Vam Asi. 'I am the Other'. Otherwise you might as well just come by looking in the mirror all day."

Nim sinks all the way under the water for a whole minute and when he comes up he spits a big mouthful of water at Jack.

"I am the scrap!" he howls. "I am completely twisted up with the whole Universe!"

†

## SUNNY

Mack's messed up about it. I'm not a psychiatrist, but I'm a pretty good nurse. Maybe not as perfect as Brandy; she had 100% perfect scores and I only got 96%. We had the same teacher, Dr. Jain, but maybe she took the assignments a little more seriously by sleeping with our patient.

After dinner Mack settles back in his office, morose and drinking bourbon.

"Watered down spritzers with dinner," he complains.

"What can I do to make things better?" I ask. "Really. There's no actual harm done."

"I've been thinking," he muses. "None of it probably matters in the end. Dave loves her. She's good for him. The marriage can't be voided unless it's contested and proven in court. Maybe we should forget about it."

"Yeah," I agree. "Except the reason it's illegal is that their children could be impaired. She should know."

"Mmm. Agreed. Incest was a pretty standard practice historically among royalty to perpetuate lineage but it produced some bad apples. She should know—nurse."

He's just handed it to me professionally. I turn it over in my head. All she really needs to know, I think, is safe sex. The complications of why she needs to keep it safe are only going to break her heart. I can do this.

I tuck Jack in bed and he seems resigned without his parents but he grumbles a little that sex isn't supposed to take *that* long. Trouble doesn't take that long, I tease him, but love does.

In the morning Dave shows up with Sim to take Jack out to play in the forest. Dave looks perfectly groomed and stunning and he takes the lead in organizing shakes for everyone.

Sim looks absolutely messed up, spaced out and lost. He keeps looking back over his shoulder like he wants to go home, but he cheers up a little when Jack comes downstairs.

While the boys are drinking breakfast, I go next door to talk to Nicky. She's sprawled on the big sofa by the gym, drinking coffee with Nat in the sunshine on the lawn. I'm relieved to have Nat there to help me with this so I can use her as leverage to bridge the subject.

"It's fun having Jack here," I start. "Lots of responsibility, but nice. I guess we need to figure out a plan to home school him. He must be a fourth-grader now."

"I'd like to help, Sunny," Nat says. "Of course Brandy will want to organize it but she's got a lot of good teachers here to help her."

"How about you, Nat?" I grab my chance. "Now that you're married, are you and Dr. Jain planning to have kids?"

"No plans," she smiles, "but we're being safe. If we do, it won't be an accident."

"Nicky?" I say ask casually, but this is really where I'm trying to drive the conversation.

"Kamadev is my baby. Why would I want another one? Anyway he's keeping me very, very busy. I had no idea he was so talented. The boy could make a fortune as a professional stripper."

"So you're taking precautions?"

"What? It's not necessary. Dave doesn't do it that way." She looks to Nat for affirmation. "He doesn't—um, come. I mean he comes a lot! But just orgasms, not insemination. That's safe isn't it?"

I wait for Nat. I don't want to seem too pushy about this.

"It's not bullet-proof, Nicky," she says. "I mean, even if he's practicing conservation of his seminal fluids, there might be a leak. If you really don't want kids, it doesn't hurt to take some extra care when you're ovulating. At least track that so you're aware."

"Oh," she says. "How do I track it? Do I have to count days?"

"The simplest way is to track your basal body temperature, right Sunny?" Now I can step in as a nurse without her suspecting my motives.

"Right. Just take your temperature in the morning. It rises and falls during the month according to your fertility. I can explain the details if you'd like. It doesn't hurt to know what's going on in your body. It's *your* body and knowledge is power."

"Fine," she grins. "Go ahead and teach me. One baby boy is all I can handle."

There, I think smugly. Solved it. She doesn't want kids, she's willing to learn how to prevent kids and no one needs to know the gritty dirty details.

Knowledge is power but ignorance is bliss.

†

## S&M

When we finish playing in the pond, Kama Dave decides to take the afternoon off work to teach Jack how to swim. We get some scissors from Sunny and cut the legs off his little jeans. She frowns because we're mutilating his new clothes but the boy needs something to swim in more than he needs jeans. Just for sport, I cut the sleeves off his little t-shirt, too, so we can watch his tiny biceps grow.

Me, I feel hungry as a wolf, relaxed and ready to try out the God of Love's disappearing theory. As soon as I get home and shut the pool house door behind me, I step out of my sweat pants and head for the yoga deck. She better be out there where I left her, behaving.

I'm as hard as a rock but I give my erection a firm friendly handshake as I walk out the back door naked in all my morning glory. I'm on fire.

Brandy is sitting on the futon in a sarong—with Nat. Uh huh. They both take a permanent impression of my construction with such unabashed appreciation, I wonder if I should set up a tip jar.

My beautiful assistant Nat has seen me naked dozens of times on the massage table, but not in my current state of arousal. Her eyes are huge and she bites down hard on the tip of her tongue.

"Good morning, boss," she stammers.

"Yeah, it's pretty good, isn't it?" I sneer at her.

I nod politely and sit down on the wooden deck boards. It's pointless to get dressed so I simply fold my legs nicely over my equipment in Siddha-Asana, the yogi adept position.

"Um. Excuse me," she starts. "Brandy wanted to talk to me. Er, wanted me to talk to you."

"And?" I ask. "Obviously I've got things going on. What's up?" And then I can't help but roar with laughter because *I'm* up so hard I have to adjust my right foot to keep it down.

"Oh, God," she moans.

"Yes? I'm listening," I tease her.

"Just one minute, boss. I just wanted to make sure you're okay, honey. How do you feel?"

I give her an evil leer. How can I answer the poor girl? Feel me? I just let the question roll around in her head until she turns scarlet.

"Please, boss," she begs. I love to hear her beg so much that I quit harassing her for a bit.

"We were worried. You were unconscious for six hours and stopped breathing. We called Rick over to check on you. Brandy said you didn't seem to know who you were or who she was when you woke up."

"Oh, that," I sneer. "That was damn good. I was really good, too, wasn't I, Brandy baby? I was smoking."

"So you know who you are now? Who are you?" Nat tests me.

"Steven S&M Fucking Mack," I growl at her. "AKA Sim, Nim, Shiva Nataraj, Sam, Dad Baby and Hey You. Who the fuck do you think I am? Did I miss anyone?"

"It sounds pretty crowded in there," she laughs nervously. "You forgot 'Boss'."

"No. I didn't forget anything. Tat Vam Asi. I am All of That. They are just names. The names dissolve into Nirvana like a candle being blown out. I'm my wife. I'm my own Mother. I might be you too, little Tantrika, if you don't watch out."

I take hold of her with my eyes and start pulling her into my solar plexus through my heart. For a brief second her eyes roll back and then she looks frightened.

"Shit, Sim. Easy, boss," she gasps and jumps up to her feet. "He's fine, Brandy. A little bit incendiary, but fine. Handle with caution, okay?"

Then she regains her equanimity and before she goes, she leaves me with some words of clear Tantric wisdom.

"Pain is your best friend, Sim, more honest than pleasure. When you can look pain in the eye your humanity disintegrates, your personality shatters and—when you submit—you open the doorway to becoming a great being."

†

## BRANDY

"Remember the night Kamadev blew his fuse on Nat?" Sim asks after she leaves. "He just disappeared on us."

How could I forget? Dave went from being a neurotic junkie virgin to a psychotic love god in a heartbeat.

Sim clamps both my wrists in his big hands like manacles and squeezes, pulling my arms around his waist.

"It's okay, baby," he purrs. "I trust you now. I've got it all figured out now. Psycho Dave explained everything to me."

I almost choke on my laugh but he puts his mouth over mine with a lovely deep kiss and then whispers his secret.

"He didn't know who the fuck he was, baby. He was lost and confused and trying to kill himself. He was so stoned on heroin, morphine, codeine and god knows what else, he was in so much pain it was only natural for him to let it all go. Just like Nat said, he disintegrated. He was forced to surrender.

"And now Jack is just as lost. His mother is dead, he doesn't even know me, he's living with a houseful of strangers and lunatics, and he's got nothing left to lose. He's just beautiful. He's so full of love it's adorable. I don't want to ruin that for him.

"I want to be him," he sighs and pushes himself into me. He's got it figured out all right. He moves like a big beautiful mountain lion.

"What you did to me, baby," he sighs, "what Nat taught you to do, you turned me loose. I'm so far gone I'm not coming back. Can you tell, honey? The whole Universe is combusting."

I can hear him talking but the words fade into colored lights and it sounds like he's singing to me now, deep and beautiful gravelly blues, singing into my mouth, singing down my spine and into my heartbeat and out through my fingers as I touch the hard muscles rocking and rolling through his back.

I feel him in me and on me and around me, flowing through me back out into his own body. He's got it all figured out so well that there's no separation between us, no space at all left. I am him. I am the Great Dancer now, the Nataraj and I spin so hard, I make the whole Universe come.

†

JACK

We never even stop for lunch. By the time Dad comes out to the pool, Uncle Dave has taught me a nice crawl stroke and I try hard to kick neatly under the water. He says don't make big crashing kicks that waste energy.

My Uncle says that my father is a great surfer and I can't learn to surf if I can't swim, so that's all I care about now. I want to be just like Dad and Uncle Kama Dave. I want to *be* them. They have big muscles and beautiful wives who give them love instead of trouble.

Dad sits down on a lawn chair to watch me swim. He's wearing a sarong because he is so famous but he laughs at Dave, "Hey brother, if it weren't for Sunny I could walk around naked all day. Every other female up here has seen it all."

"It's not the women you need to worry about, Nim," Uncle snorts. "Prince would have a heart attack. It's probably not polite either, especially at the table."

"Hmmpf," he grunts happily. He's not so serious now. He looks free like Uncle Kama Dave. "Chef's day off!" he laughs, unties the sarong and stretches out on his stomach on the lawn like a big happy dog.

I get out of the pool and sit on the grass next to him, just to stare. He has so many muscles and lines and scars on his back that he looks like his own puzzle. It looks like terrible trouble. I stare at Dad's back and Uncle watches me staring.

"Does it hurt?" I ask and put my finger on one of the marks carefully.

"Nah," my father says. "It's my best friend."

†

## DJ

Everything is going perfectly on top of our world right now even without Prince to fix us lunch. Then all of a sudden the whole Universe starts to unravel with a blood-curdling roar.

I hear the tremendous thunder of a big motorcycle engine coming up the mountain from a mile away and then dead silence. A couple minutes later, the peace is broken again by a piercing wolf whistle as Billy Lee comes around the side of the house.

"Oh, the bad boys are at it again," he hoots, and he looks pretty wrecked. I can feel his vibration even more clearly than I can see it—I know the taste of it. Heroin.

"Nim!" I hiss a warning and he lifts his head up from the grass to take a look.

"Shit, Billy!" he swears.

"Sam, old buddy, S&M!" Billy howls. "My old friend. You wild man! You better throw some clothes over yourself, buddy. My girl is coming just behind me.

"Wait til you see this one! She's atomic. Filthy rich. She bought me the bike, man. Lots of candy, too. I've struck pay dirt, baby! My sugar momma!"

Nim ties the sarong back on and gives Billy a menacing glare.

"Candy?" he snarls. "You've got balls coming up here loaded, Billy Boy."

"Is that any way to treat your old friend, Sammy? My girl wanted to meet you. Heard all about you, bro.

"Here she comes, what did I say? She can strike a man blind."

Billy's 'girl' is nearly twice as old as me. She struts over to Nim and holds out her hand, loaded with jewelry, with rocks big enough to anchor a little boat.

She's very beautiful and built like Nicky with all the womanly parts you'd ever want to see but she looks mean. She looks brutally mean. She looks at Nim very suggestively and purrs hello into his neck. Then she turns to me looking like she's going to bite my head off and have fun doing it.

She's dressed in skin tight black stretchy stuff that shows everything, pointy shiny leather boots and a soft little fur vest zipped down low. Venus in furs, worse than Kali, worse than my old nightmares. And then I realize I know her. Mother Fuck! She's the one who threw me away. Mommy!

"Sammy, meet Diana," Billy growls.

"FUCK!" I scream and run like hell for my room.

†

## S&M

"Who the hell is that rude little bastard?" Diana demands. "Impudent little fucker."

"Don't worry about him, babe," Billy apologizes. "He's mentally ill. But he's not that dumb. He uh, married your sister."

"Billy tells me you know my sister," she interrupts him. "Her famous rich boyfriend. I've been looking for her for weeks but her place is deserted. She married that little prick? I don't get it."

She looks me up and down concentrating on my chest and the scars on my abs and then really staring at my sarong like she's trying to measure the size of my equipment. She gives me the chills and I wish I had my leathers on right now for my own protection.

"He's my brother," I hiss and Billy's jaw drops. It's news to him. He's been out of the picture for months.

"Does that make you my rich brother in law then instead of her rich boyfriend?" she teases.

I look at her closely and I can see the resemblance and I'm even more furious with Billy for bringing her up than I am for reintroducing me to his drug habit. This is our sanctuary, our retreat and Nicky despises her big sister.

"Jack baby," I say, "why don't you go home and let Sunny give you a bath. I'll be over later."

He's already heard things I wish he hadn't. He gives me the little okay mudra and takes off.

I don't want to give her any more information about us, but I'm afraid Billy has already said a lot.

So I just play it cool, cold as ice. I put an arm around Billy and walk him a few steps away from her as if I'm his best friend. I was. I guess I still am even though I'd like to nail him into the ground right now. I lower my voice so she can't hear and I'll bet $500 she thinks we're talking about how hot she is.

"I hear Sean's got his eye on you, Mr. Lee," I say. "He's threatening to bring you up here the hard way. You know what that means. Arrest, man."

Billy's face turns white and he stammers. "No, man. I can't do that. I'm not like you and Dave. I can't be tied down, restrained in one place. It's nice here, but I gotta come and go. That doesn't work for me."

"Sean wouldn't be happy to hear I saw you hammered, Billy. I might not say anything if you promise to keep a low profile.

"Nicky doesn't want to see her sister, you know what I mean? Women can be—territorial, you know."

"I just thought you'd dig her, Sam. She's hot, don't you think?"

"She's scorching hot, Billy. Don't burn yourself. But you know Nicky. Even though she's married, she's pretty jealous of me. She wouldn't understand. Why don't you show me that new motorcycle the lady bought you?"

I don't care what it looks like, it's just a smooth way to get them out of my yard and off my property. He relaxes a little and calls her. "Come on, babe. Sammy wants to see the new bike."

We walk around the house and Billy sneers in my ear, "Ya got no idea how much I put out in trade for this toy, Sam man!"

Besides sex? I wonder. Besides stabbing his old buddy in the back by telling her who I am and showing her where I live? I have a pretty good idea she's been using him to find us but no clue why.

I give enough time and attention to the hot wheels to stoke Billy's ego and I even smooth it over a little with Diana. So I don't offend her, I ask for her phone number and she gushes all over me.

"If I see Nicky, I'll have her call you," I lie.

She asks for my number and I tell her truthfully I don't have a phone. All our lines are unlisted, restricted to business. Ah, the joy of the Corporate veil. I don't own anything. As the CEO, I just have shares.

I'm smirking, very pleased with how smoothly I handled her, until she puts a hand on my arm and asks urgently, "How about the Doctor?"

"What doctor?" I ask innocently. We have two after all.

"You've got another brother don't you? Very much older, in his fifties. Dr. Mack. I need to talk to him urgently. It's a private matter."

"Huh?" I stammer. Mack just looks old. He's younger than she is. I'm keeping him out of this.

"He's a very busy man," I say. "You'll need an appointment. But I'll give your number to his secretary and have her set one up."

What in hell kind of business can she have with Mack? As they drive off down the mountain, I watch the sun settling into the far-off bank of fog rolling over the ocean. And I watch the darkness creeping up the mountain.

†

## NICK

It's late afternoon and I'm sitting at the boardroom table with Nat having a glass of wine. It's the chef's day off so we're not getting the watered-down spritzers today; we've broken into one of his vintage Pinot Noirs.

Dave's been giving the kid swimming lessons while S&M was busy with transcendental sex lessons, so it's been a peaceful day in the Fire House. The only problem we have is whether to make a healthy Ayurvedic kitchari for dinner or order Mexican takeout.

We're leaning towards some more wine and the takeout when we hear the side door slam, footsteps pounding up the stairs and then the upstairs door slam.

I go to the bottom of the stairs and call "Kama Dave? Is that you, honey?" but there's no answer. When I go up the door's locked. I can hear water running but nobody answers. I pound pretty hard, but get nothing.

"What's his problem?" I complain to Nat and pour another glass. "He was in a beautiful mood all day. Do we have a key for that door?"

She sighs. "We've got the window locked from the inside and probably should have had the door locked from the outside. I thought he was well now."

S&M comes through the kitchen looking tanned and beautiful but furious. He smirks at the bottle of wine and goes back to the kitchen for another glass.

"Bitch!" he swears as he throws one down and pours another looking around. "Where's Kamadev? She scared the piss out of him. He probably needs a drink."

"I think he's locked himself in the bedroom, baby," I say. "Having a bath. I don't really know. He won't let me in. Who scared him?"

"Your sister Diana," he hisses. "Billy Lee is her new boy toy. And you know Billy. He's all about the money and she's loaded. I can't believe he brought her up here."

"She's been looking for me, baby. Sean brought me a letter yesterday saying she was desperate for money and some other crap about getting a fortune from some man."

He flinches. "Where's the letter?"

"I asked Sean to burn it, but I think Mack picked it up. Is she gone?"

"Yeah, yeah, don't worry, honey. I said you weren't here. But fucking Billy told her Dave is your husband. She's freaking me out. What's her game?"

"Same as Billy I guess. Same as ever, looking for easy money."

"I'll handle it, Nicky," he promises. "I'll fucking handle everything."

He finishes the second glass and goes upstairs while we wait. It's impossible not to hear it. Knocking then pounding; orders followed by curses then threats.

"Fucking open the door right now, little brother before I kick it down. You will not like it if I have to break the door down, Fucker! I will lock you up for a week in the nurses' room with no toys, no food and no sex!"

When he comes back down he points to his empty glass and I can almost see smoke coming out of his ears.

"He's not talking, but he turned the water off to listen so he's not dead. Fuck! Who's got a key?"

"Let me call Rick," Nat says. "He must have one."

But before she picks up the phone, Brandy comes in through the kitchen. She's got her big hypodermic needle and ampules of lorazepam.

"Sunny authorized it," she says. "Dave called me."

"You talked to him?" S&M wonders. "What did he say?"

"He called me 'Mommy'. He said only I can come in because he's hiding. Let me take care of him, baby. I'm his nurse. He'll be fine."

S&M sinks into the chair speechless. When Brandy goes upstairs and doesn't come back, he exhales a big sigh.

"Nicky baby, let's go see Mack," he mutters.

†

MACK

Sunny is upstairs playing with Jack and his wails of laughter are tickling me while I try to concentrate on business. I wonder if she could ever make me scream with pleasure like that. Cold day in hell, I think.

When Steven and Nicky appear at the office door I wonder what took them so long. I tried to warn her yesterday. Now I'm not so sure I want to.

"Steven," I start. He winces. "Brother," I correct myself. "We should have a word in private."

"There's nothing you can say to me that you can't say in front of my girl," he says smugly.

"Try me," I challenge him.

He narrows his eyes and frowns, but he sits down on the big couch and crosses his legs under him. "Nicky, sweetheart, get lost. I'm handling this."

"Thank you," I sigh with relief as she closes the door behind her. "I'll tell her everything if you want, but you should think about it first."

"She said there's a letter," he muses. "From Diana."

"The letter she got yesterday is pretty tame, brother. What she doesn't know about is the letter I got a few weeks ago. I just didn't know who the hell Diana was until she showed me hers."

I take the older letter out of my desk and pass it to him and let him drink it in. He looks at me in shock while he does the math.

"Dad could have a lot of 21 year old kids," I reason, "but Diana can only have one. Who's to say which one he is?"

I pass him the bourbon but he pushes it away. "Who's to say?" I repeat. "Do you really want to pursue this?"

"I'm not the one pursuing it, Mack," Steven whines hopelessly. "She is. She was here today. She's looking for Dad isn't she?"

"I think so. Look, I'm willing to meet with her and explain that Dad passed away 15 years ago. We don't owe her anything since she abandoned her kid. Whether it was Dave or some other kid, does it matter?

"Think about this, Steven." He's no longer flinching at the sound of his name. He's beyond that. "She put her kid in a foster home. She doesn't know he's here."

"No. She didn't recognize him. He was only 6. But I bet he recognized her. She probably hasn't changed much in 15 years. But he ran away before she introduced herself."

"We could easily wade through this shit, little brother. I'll get rid of Diana and get the fox out of the henhouse and all will be well with the world.

"What Nicky doesn't know won't hurt her. Think about that very hard, brother. I wish I didn't know what I know.

"Dave doesn't know Diana is Nicky's sister. Nicky doesn't know Dave is Diana's son. And Diana doesn't know anything! Let's keep it that way."

Steven pulls the bourbon back again and drinks straight out of the bottle.

"Dave and Nicky, shit," he groans. "This is worse than me and Nicky. You're right, brother. You'd wish you didn't know what I know!"

"Trust me, Steven. Sometimes compassion becomes more important than truth. No one else knows except Sunny and she's very discreet. She's already talked to Nicky about preventing any, um complications."

"Kids? Oh, that. Fuck!" he laughs. "I'd like to see someone try to draw that twisted family tree."

†

DJ

Only her. My real mother. Only she can see me. When I flew through the window I swallowed all of the glass and I can feel all the broken sharp edges of it inside me now. If I cough or move, the pieces of it will spit up and cut me. I can taste it.

It's better if I sit in the silky water and float. Nim screams and screams but I can't tell him about all the broken glass inside me. Only her.

When I hear the quiet tapping, I put the saffron golden silk kimono on and whisper at the door. "Mother?"

"Yes, Baby Dave," she says. "I'm here."

I open the door and she has the nice needle and caring eyes and I will be safe in here now. I let her in and lock the door again.

"Lie down, baby," she says, but I explain to her that I'm full of glass and it might cut me if I lie down. I have to float in the water.

"Glass?" she wonders.

"Yes," I tell her patiently. "All the broken edges and sharp pointy pieces are inside me. Everything will cut me if I lie down."

"Not if you lie down with me," she promises. "Carefully. I'll make sure nothing breaks inside you."

She helps me carefully onto the bed and nothing breaks and she holds her arms around me and puts her hands over my eyes and sings a nice little song.

"See?" she smiles. "Everything is fine. Would you like a shot, baby?"

"Yes please, mom."

"The shot will take all the glass away. Would you like to tell me how you flew through the window?"

She pulls the sleeve of the kimono up and finds my beautiful veins, nice clean veins since I've been lifting weights instead of shooting dope. Fine. Fine. I feel the psychotics flowing into my blood like a nice wine and all the glass starts to melt.

Then I open my eyes and explain everything to her. I show her my knuckles with the pretty Om tattoo that reminds me of milky oceans and sexy snakes.

"This line," I point, "the crescent underneath the dot, is the window. Everything is dancing in front of the window. But behind the window, the dot is hiding. That's me. I broke through the glass and I'm hiding there."

"I think Nim is there, too," she whispers. "He's very lonely. Would you talk to him?"

"Only you, mom. Nim is very angry. I would not like to see him break the door down and lock me up."

"Why did you fly through the window, baby?" she wonders. I would rather not tell her about the bad mother, the one who wanted to bite my head off and throw me away again.

"I'm not a baby," I sneer. "Sometimes a man just feels like disintegrating."

"Oh. Fine. Fine," she purrs. She strokes my forehead and I close my eyes so I can watch the screen inside my head and the candle burning in the darkness behind my third eye. I hear her counting my body parts. Right thumb, right index finger, right middle finger... and before she even gets to my elbow I fall completely and perfectly inside myself.

†

## PRINCE ALBERT

They've gone through three bottles of our best Pinot Noir and have another one open. I was saving it for a special roast lamb dinner. I've just bought a case of vintage Cabernet Sauvignon and I'm tempted to lock it up in my room. That's a chef's plight. As fast as I can buy food and wine, they consume it. And eventually it all turns to shit.

S&M, Nicky and Nat are throwing dice, each without their respective partners. You'd expect they'd be feeling pretty happy but they're dismal. No one had lunch or dinner. No one cooked or ordered takeout.

When I walk in, they all give me the psycho lost look that Dave does so well. It gives me a little thrill of pleasure to see the hopeless gloom hanging over the boardroom table. They need me. They really need me.

They're not playing for money and they're not playing strip dice. Apparently they're just playing for points, playing for the Game. It's the darkest joyless play I've ever seen at the gaming table.

Nat explains that Dave is ill, Brandy is taking care of him, and Dr. Jain is upstairs taking the lock off the bedroom door. I wonder if Dave's strip act got out of control. I don't want to know.

"Hungry?" I suggest. It's my day off but they look pitiful. I know I'll get another raise for this.

S&M bought me 'French Country Cooking' after he split my head open for dealing dope. In it Elizabeth David wrote that a good omelette and a fine vintage is the most primitive and elemental meal. They've already got the vintage open and they look desperately primitive. It's a match made in heaven.

"Omelettes?" I offer.

"Hell, yes! Where have you been all my life?" S&M teases drunkenly. He gets up from the table seriously and drops down on his knees. "Will you marry me? Say yes, Prince honey."

Any other day that would have horrified me, but he looks terribly hungry and beaten down in spite of his smile. I can see it's just a joke, an act, and the ladies are laughing in sympathy.

"You can't afford me," I snort smugly. "Just the food for now."

He laughs like a drowning man catching some air and I suspect I've missed a lot of trouble today. I don't even know my boss. I've been too frightened to look at him.

But now that I'm looking I can see he's fighting for breath and reason, fighting to keep his head above water like a desperate junkie and fighting to keep his little brother's head above water. Ouch. I'm sorry I ever called Dave his little bitch.

He winks at me and bows his head submissively as if I've just crushed him with my rejection. That causes another round of laughs and I join in too.

I pick up the score pad for the dice game and start taking orders. Cheese, mushrooms, chilis, olives, chives, tarragon, thyme, and everyone wants everything. I want to give everyone everything.

I watch the room warm up with light and gratitude. I'm happy to be home again.

When I start serving the plates, I get more marriage proposals from Nicky and Nat. Everyone is having a good joke.

"Sorry," I smirk. "No, thank you."

Dr. Jain has joined the table now with the disassembled bedroom doorknob on the table in front of him. He's missed out on the joke, but as I hand him his plate, I say, "No thanks, I'm already taken."

The rest of them howl with joy at the doctor's confused look. Then, last of all, I hand S&M the best omelette of my life and—do I dare?—I wink at him and quickly retreat to the privacy of my kitchen.

I can hardly breathe. I don't want to eat. That was my best service ever, simple omelettes. I sneak a glass of red wine for myself and sit down at the kitchen counter to catch my breath. I'm proud of it.

Then I hear it, applause and shouts of 'encore', like a good rock'n roll band finale. And they don't quit! I feel my face turning the color of the wine but finally I come out and bow and start collecting the dishes and a few kisses as the ladies give me a standing ovation.

When I finish cleaning the kitchen and go to my room they're back to playing dice seriously. Apparently Brandy is sleeping with Dave. I'll never understand these people.

It's after 11 by the time I shower and dress in my pajama pants. I've missed a dozen texts from Cat: teasing texts, joking texts, demanding texts and finally whining texts. I turn the phone off again and stare into the mirror.

I wish my hair were dark like his. It's just plain dirty blond. I wish my eyes were blue or green instead of muddy brown. I wonder how a little chain around my neck would look. But finally I crawl under the sheets, close my eyes and wait for sleep.

And then I can't stop seeing him on his knees in front of everyone: the most powerful man I know, the richest, the kindest and the toughest, on his knees in front of me with his head hanging down in despair. A man with a beautiful wife, a gorgeous girlfriend and a hundred children on his knees in front of me.

I reach my hand out and touch the crown of his head. I pet his black hair and he looks up at me with surprised blue eyes. And I say 'Yes'.

†

NICK

It's after midnight when Nat and Jain go to bed so I come outside with S&M to stare at the stars. We're lying on the lumpy old sofa bed on the lawn by the gym, my head on his shoulder but nothing else touching.

It's easy. We spent six years being intimate without touching each other and now even this, lying against his shoulder, is closer than we used to come. I have a powerful sense of him as my protector. More than a boyfriend or a sugar daddy, he's my big brother now. He'll handle everything.

It's a moonless night and everything is in Technicolor: pulsing red, pink, yellow and blue stars, dusty silver celestial clouds and occasional satellites creeping across the sky.

He doesn't speak at all; his breath is long and slow, calmly mulling over the state of the Universe. After a long while he reaches down and squeezes my hand.

"Go to bed, Nick," he whispers. "I've got this."

From the tone of his voice, I'm convinced he has the entire Cosmos tucked safely in his back pocket. Every bit of Divine perfection has been carefully laid in place within the puzzle and now it's his watch. Nothing can go wrong. I kiss his forehead and go back to the house.

Upstairs Dave is curled up in a little ball in the middle of the bed. He's got Brandy's fingertips clamped in his fist and the back of his hand pressed to his mouth. I crawl in quietly behind him and put my hand on his heart and fall into dreamless sleep.

In the morning, I hear him wake. "Oh," he says looking at Brandy. "Oh." And then he rolls over and sees me. "Oh! I'm hungry," he says as if nothing happened. "Can we have breakfast? I have to go to work."

†

## S&M

Me, I'm handling everything. I watch the stars until they fade into the dawn's light and there's nothing left but the morning planet Venus. Then I get up and stretch into a rhythmic Surya Namaskar, the Sun Salutation.

I can feel the prana of starlight gathered in the dew of the wet morning lawn. I feel it drawing up from the ground through my bare feet, up my spine and out through my fingertips as I reach up to bless the world.

With every inhale I draw the life force from the earth through my feet. With every exhale I pour it back out over the top of the world. Om Namah Shivaya. I redistribute all the fallen stardust on the mountaintop to the rest of the world. By the time the sun rises, the planet is well blessed and nicely sorted.

Prince is busy in the Fire House kitchen when I return to the rich smell of dark coffee. He gives me a fleeting glance with a strange smirk as if a smile might cause him pain.

"Would you rather have black tea?" he asks.

"Don't bother. I'm easy," I tease. "I go both ways."

His mouth gapes and he blushes deeply.

"Oh, come on!" I admonish him. "Lighten up man. Coffee or tea. It's a joke. Coffee's fine."

I take my cup into the boardroom so he can relax in his own space. Man, the kid is wired tighter than a time bomb!

A few minutes later he follows me with the pot and tops my cup off. “Sorry,” he mumbles. “I didn’t mean to—”

“To insinuate?” I laugh. “Breathe, man. You really ought to learn how to breathe.”

He stands there nervously looking at me, and takes a deep breath, but he forgets to exhale. So I demonstrate with a big gusty ‘HAH!’ I finally get a smile from him but still he won’t make eye contact.

“Look,” I say, making a concerted effort not to call him ‘honey’. I wait until he actually looks me square in the eye.

“I’m sorry that we teased you last night, but you were brilliant. I don’t really know how to show you my appreciation without embarrassing or offending you.

And then I take the first step down that twisted road of the human heart. “No offense, man. But we all love you.”

For a split second I see a flash of joy and wonder in his eyes and then he shuts everything down and all the lights go off. I change the subject to try and lighten him back up.

“Do you know you can control your body with your breath? You can change your heart rate and blood pressure and even your temperature.”

He squints at me like I’m from another planet, but I go on.

“Part of yoga is simple breathing. It’s called Pranayama. Prana is your life force and energy, and Pranayama, breath control, teaches you how to change your energy using your breath. Cool, huh?”

“I’ve got to start breakfast,” he says mechanically. “What are you having?”

“Duh!” I joke. “I’m having the rock star omelette again. Whatdya think? But first you have to humor your boss. Sit down and try this or you’re fired.”

He sits at the table and pours me some more coffee but I can't read him. It's as if he's not really here or not sure if he really wants to be here. He's more disconcerting than Dave, more tentative. There's only a very slender thread connecting him to the present.

"Okay," I instruct, "you're going to use your thumb and ring finger like this." I show him how to alternate between the two to close either the right or left nostril with the first two fingers lightly resting on his third eye for steadiness.

He tries it and laughs, "It's silly!"

"Yeah, yogi queer stuff," I joke. "Humor me."

Then I show him how to count his breath. He's young so I use an eight count. In through the left, out through the right; in through the right, out through the left. Ten rounds at one per minute, we breathe together for ten minutes. Time stops. I'm watching his eyes turn from muddy brown to bright gold. I'm watching all the lights turn on.

I don't even have to ask him how he feels when he's done. I can see it. He's gazing into my eyes like he belongs there. He's letting himself be seen. His feet are connected to the earth and his head is connected to the stars.

"Smooth," I remark.

"Yeah. Man. Smooth. Very. Smooth," he smiles.

He sits there just looking at me without flinching, without blinking, looking at me like maybe he knows me.

"Hey," I say, "When we brought you up here to the ICU I thought you were a red head. But it was just all the fucking blood on you. I'm truly sorry. I lost my temper. I'm really not in the habit of abducting minors. You were my first."

It's meant to be a joke but it fails miserably and I see his eyes darken. He may be the first kid I assaulted but it wasn't the first time for him. The uneasiness, the defensiveness and the fear aren't all directed at me. He's been repeatedly abused, scared to death and traumatized.

His profession is his act, a safe appearance in this world. When he was the regional heroin sales manager, he had structure and safety. Now his only excuse for being present is as my personal chef. Otherwise, I think he'd run for the hills.

I want to put my arm around him and tell him how clearly I see him, how perfectly welcome he is to be alive on this planet, but all I've ever managed to offer him was another raise or another round of praise. I don't even think the money matters as much to him as he thinks, except as a badge of honor and worth.

"Would you mind?" I venture. "Could I have that omelette?"

"Same as last night?" he lights up, raising a questioning eyebrow.

"Never," I laugh. "Never repeat yourself, buddy. Use your imagination."

He laughs like a man grateful for the air, like a reprieved criminal. "You've got it, honey," he smirks in a perfect impersonation of me.

As he gets up from the table he puts his hand on my back. He puts his hand right behind my heart and nearly melts it.

†

## PRINCE ALBERT

I put more intention and attention into this omelette than anything I've ever cooked, carefully whisking the eggs with pink Himalayan salt, tri-colored cracked peppercorns, and finely diced tarragon and thyme as I heat the sweet butter to a perfect foamy simmer.

I stir in the eggs, let them set and at just the right moment I add chopped mushrooms and chives tossed in fig vinegar and roll it carefully onto a plate. It's an insane omelette but the smell is intoxicating. When I set it down in front of him, I can almost taste my laurels and I wait for the accolades.

Instead of digging into it, he looks up at the stairs where crazy Dave is standing nervously, frozen in his tracks, dressed in nothing but his ratty old jeans. We haven't seen *those* in a while. His wife and his nurse are following behind him, waiting for him to take another step.

"What's wrong with him?" I ask impatiently.

"Nothing much," he says. "Probably air sickness. Sometimes he just forgets to breathe."

S&M raises his hand and beckons to Dave with a curled finger.

"Come on down, baby brother. I didn't mean to shout at you. I was really mad at Billy. I'm sorry."

Dave takes a few cautious steps down as if he's walking into a trap. When S&M gets to his feet, he actually takes a step back up a stair and bumps into Brandy.

"Come on, Kamadev," S&M purrs. "I was wrong. I'm not angry. Come on and have breakfast."

He puts his arms out and when Dave finally gets to the table he gives him a bear hug. I feel my blood drain and a chill in my toes. Shit, I'm jealous. And the eggs are getting cold!

How does Dave get away with this? He's been sleeping with two women and then he gets a hug! And as he sits down at the table S&M gives him his omelette! All the love I put into that special breakfast and he just gives it away.

"Hey, Prince, can you make a few more?" he says.

I've lost my place in his attention now as he busies himself with his wife, his girl friend and his brother. I lift my chin and pretend I don't care and head back to the kitchen infuriated.

How can I make three more all that special? How would I know which one is his? How can everything be special? I start cracking the eggs in misery but he comes back into the kitchen.

"Hey, man, can you make a frittata?" he wonders.

"Of course I can," I hiss making a face at him like he was born yesterday. I'd really like to hit him. I wonder how he got the black eye.

"Well, look. Make that then instead, one big frittata for everyone, family style. And then come and sit down and eat with us, man."

He puts his hand on my shoulder and smiles at me so sweetly I want to kiss him now. I wonder if he will ever hug me. I'm getting horribly mixed up now, afraid he's really getting serious and at the same time afraid he really doesn't care.

I look in his eyes, one at a time and see nothing but kindness. I don't think he'll hurt me again. I'm on his side. But I'm worried. What if he really does love me? What will he do? How can he make love to four different people? What would even happen?

Then I remember what I told him last night. Just the food for now. Anything more is just too complicated. I don't even want to know about it.

†

## NAT

Jain leaves at dawn for the hospital and by the time I get up there are already five of them sitting around the boardroom table for breakfast. It's very odd to see Prince sitting with them.

Kama Dave eats like a starving boy, nearly inhaling his omelette and then diving ravenously into the frittata. He's not talking to anyone but he's behaving carefully. Normally, he'd be spoon-feeding Nicky but he ignores everyone except for an occasional nervous glance at Sim.

"You kno-o-w, brother," Sim finally drawls, "I want my wife back. She's not your mother."

Dave makes a horrible face like he's being robbed at gunpoint and sniffs hard.

"You don't need a mother, honey," he continues. "*I* don't have a mother. Mack doesn't have a mother. Prince here doesn't have a mother, right honey?" he turns to his chef who's sitting beside him for a change, staring at him with fascination. Prince shakes his head compliantly like an obedient pet.

"You're just fine without a mother," Sim repeats. "You don't have to have one." I don't understand what's going on between them but it sounds like a promise of protection is being made. Dave lets out a deep sigh of relief.

"I've got you, baby," Sim continues. "I'll handle it. Right now, I'm going over to see Mack and I'll take care of everything.

"Nat?" he instructs me, "Put him to work but stay out of this."

As he gets up to leave, Prince jumps to his feet to start clearing the table. Sim puts his hand on Prince's back and whispers something but I can't hear what he says. Prince nods a little vacantly and takes the plates back to the kitchen.

"I'm more worried about that one, Nat," he says seriously. "He could definitely use a little therapy if you have some time."

I decide to kill two birds with one stone when the boss leaves with the women. I offer to help Prince clean the kitchen if he helps us in the lab.

"No, thanks," he sneers. "I have shopping and prep. S&M needs me."

I look at him carefully and see exactly what the boss is worried about. He's too rigid and obsessive about his role in the household, frightened, anxious and precariously unstable. But I see a big chink in his thick armor and I aim for it.

"Sim asked me to show you some things you might be able to use," I say. Nicer than saying your boss said you can use some therapy.

"Um, what kind of stuff?" he asks nervously. He's never set foot in the lab.

"Just some simple stuff. How we use plants to create balance, like you do with food. It doesn't hurt to learn."

"Mmm," he thinks. "He said he wants me to learn? He taught me some prawn stuff this morning."

"Pranayama," Dave sniffs condescendingly. "Breath control."

"Yeah," Prince smiles a little. "It's smooth."

"Even smoother with the oils," Dave says. He pulls out his vial of lotus oil and demonstrates. I see Prince's resistance softening with curiosity.

"Better not try this one," Dave commands. "It's a love oil. Maybe you should try it with the kid's stuff."

Prince glares at him offended and then looks at me angrily.

"Come on," I say. "I'll let you try anything we've got. Anything and everything."

Now I've got two ticking time bombs in my lab but therapy is what I do best. I get Dave busy cleaning the shelves and lining up all the bottles according to their function—a real challenge because most botanicals have multiple uses.

Prince watches with amazement as Dave sorts and proclaims: sedative, energetic, sattvic, antiseptic, aphrodisiac, meditative, nervine, musculoskeletal, focus, dreaming, creativity.

"They're like ingredients for a human recipe," Prince marvels. "Can you really change the flavor of people like that, like spicing a sauce?"

"That's the idea," I say. "I knew you'd like this. The plants have energy and information that you can 'borrow' to inform your being—body, mind and spirit—by using your sense perceptions."

"But you don't drink it!" Dave laughs. "Not these. The tinctures are okay, but these are too powerful. Smell is the most basic sense so it works very well to just breathe it. The best thing to do is have a massage and get the stuff all over you."

"Nobody's touching me!" Prince bristles.

"Oh, that's funny!" Dave sneers. "'Don't look at me or talk to me or touch me!' Did Nim teach you that? That's for celibates and virgins. If you're that nervous about it, you can just rub it on yourself."

Prince blushes.

"If you know so much, Dave, why are you still psycho?" he hisses.

"Why are *you* still blonde?" Dave snorts.

I'm afraid Prince is going to put his wall back up, so I interrupt.

"Smelling is fine. There's a lot of information available through the nose. Just like in cooking. You can tell something is done baking by its smell."

I hand him one of the bottles that I know he needs right now: pure Italian bergamot oil. He sniffs it and his eyes brighten.

"Earl Grey!" he enthuses. "It's the flavor in tea! What does it do?"

"You tell me," I encourage him. "Try using it like Sim showed you. Use one side of your nose at a time."

I'm afraid that if I tell him bergamot is a nervine sedative used to calm anxiety and fears, to balance moods, he will resist my diagnosis. By regulating the hypothalamus gland it can steady unstable emotions.

I've got this boy's number. Besides hunger and body rhythms, the hypothalamus is an important regulator of emotional attachments, parenting and sexual orientation.

But experiential knowledge is much more powerful than reason, so I let him breathe and experience the effect. He works with it doing nadi shodana for two or three minutes and then he gives me a big smile.

"It makes me feel safe," he says. "I wonder—what would it do to me if I had it—in a massage?"

"Oh. Would you trust me to do that?" I'm completely surprised but then again, the oil is boosting his confidence already.

"Mmm, maybe," he says sniffing some more. "But *he* has to go."

"Before he goes, let him mix something special for you, Prince. He's very good at this."

I hand Dave the bergamot and let him smell it and he thinks about it. He picks up a bottle of tulsi, the stuff we're using on Sim for emotional scars, shows it to me and I smile. Then he picks up a bottle of laurel, which is useful for low self-esteem and doubt.

He mixes the three oils together in a glass and smells it. “Shit, *I* need this!” he exclaims.

He mixes some more, divides it into two bottles and presents one to Prince. “Rx Prince,” he laughs. “Good enough?”

“Oh. Um, thank you,” Prince stammers after smelling it and Dave walks out with a smug smile.

I take the glass and add some of it to the almond carrier oil. I put a clean sheet on the massage table and hand him one.

“I won’t look,” I promise. “Just undress and lie on your back and cover yourself with this one.”

I turn my back on him and marvel at the privilege of his trust and the chance to polish his heart and soul. His body is just a container. If Rick lays a hand on *this* one, there’s going to be a divorce.

†

## SUNNY

It’s always interesting to execute Sim’s Presidential corporate dictates, but this one is a lot more entertaining than the time he cut off the doctors’ prescriptions. Sim and I spend an hour in Mack’s office drinking tea and composing a letter, which is pure fiction but functional; then he calls Nicky and invites her over to sign it.

“How much do you trust me, honey?” he smiles as she settles in the CFO’s big office chair.

“All the way, baby,” she says without hesitation.

"Thought so," he purrs. "I'm assuming your sister wouldn't recognize your handwriting. Good. It will save you a lot of copying. Just sign it."

She signs the letter he had me write without even reading it and he looks a little surprised.

"You *can* read it, Nicky," he instructs her. "You probably *should* read it in case you need to get your story straight."

"Yes, please do, Nicky," I laugh. "It's pretty hot. Read it out loud. We might get a Pulitzer prize for this."

"Fine," she says. *"'Dear Diana. I received your letter asking for help. I wish I could but I've had some terrible luck recently. My 'rich boyfriend' turned out to be a real dick. He was shot a few months ago and married his nurse, a complete stranger. I married his little brother after that but he is a useless psychotic adolescent. I've had it with both those boys. They are selfish lunatic perverts.*

*"'I am getting a divorce and taking the next plane to Hawaii so I'll be gone by the time you get this. However, I can help you out a little bit. The rent on my beach cottage is paid in advance and it's vacant. You can stay there as long as you like or as long as the dick keeps paying the rent. I'll have a friend drop off a key for you under the mat.*

*"'I'll send you a letter when I get settled in Hawaii. Your Sister, '*

"Hang on! "She gets my house?"

"Nicky," Sim laughs, "Fuck the cottage. If we want to move back to the beach, you can live with me at my house. You're my family now, not a kept woman."

She smiles at him gratefully and giggles. "What terrible selfish lunatic perverts you boys turned out to be! I never knew you were both such pricks. But why give Diana anything? She's a piece of work."

"Nicky, I'd like Sean to keep an eye on her and Billy. This way she's just down the street from him. If they keep doing narcotics, he'll pack them away."

She nods and then looks at him in horror. "He wouldn't—um, bring them up here for rehab?"

"I don't think the board of directors would approve of that. She's trying to extort money from us. Mack and I will meet with her and deal with that.

"All you have to do is disappear when she comes up. Do you think you can handle locking yourself up in the bedroom with Dave for a day?" he smirks.

She gives him a little evil laugh. "Would you let us use the pool house, baby?"

"Sure, but don't—please, please—don't talk to Dave about this. Not a word. She really disturbed him. My guess is it's because of the narcotics," he lies. He's so cool, so slick and believable that it scares me, but I remind myself he's only lying because he cares so much about them. "Please, Nick. Don't ever mention her or any of this to him."

"Oh? Don't tell him what a useless psychotic adolescent he's turned out to be? You can trust me to trust your judgment, baby. I'll do whatever it takes. Even if it means subjecting myself to another afternoon of Kamadev's exotic floorshow."

†

JACK

Dad doesn't like Diana and I know why. Even I can see she's full of trouble instead of love. Just being beautiful isn't enough; you also have to shine. Her eyes are dark without sparkle and when she smiles she looks hungry like she wants to eat you up.

Uncle Dave gets very scared by her and even screams and then Dad makes me go home. After that, there's no fun. There's no family dinner and no bedtime stories from my mother and Aunt Nicky. Everyone is upset. Even Sunny and Mack are upset, but Sunny gives me a bath and a nice sandwich with milk in the Ice House kitchen.

I tell her about my swimming lessons and she promises to buy me some little board shorts like Dad's. I'm afraid to ask her for a sarong because I'm really not famous yet.

In the morning, there's still no mother and no Dad and no Uncle Dave to take me out to play and no shakes, just toast and milk. I blame everything on Aunt Diana for making a mess out of our house.

Sunny lets me go outside to play but makes me promise not to go down the forest trail. I peek in the window of the pool house and there's no one in there, nobody home at Dad's place, so I just sit at the edge where the lawn ends and the forest begins and hope my Fang comes up.

Nothing even happens, but I remember what Dad taught me: if you wait patiently everything will come around. I put my hands in the sign for 'patient and happy' with the thumbs on the middle fingers and smile. I trust Dad.

There's no sign of Fang but I see a lizard run past in a big hurry and some very shy little gold finches pop around me hunting for treats in the lawn. Uncle Dave sneaks up on me so quietly I don't hear him until he drops down on the grass beside me.

He doesn't look scared anymore. He grins at me and shows me a little bottle that smells like oranges and forest leaves. He's just mixed it up in the lab where he works with Nat. It's very nice.

Uncle says he's not allowed in the forest alone either so we can't go, even if we go together. He has some strong rules, too. Only with Dad or Nicky he says and they're both busy now with Uncle Mack. But we can swim before lunch!

Uncle Dave sits on the side of the pool and watches my laps, sniffing his orange oil. I swim across the width, short laps instead of long laps, in the middle of the pool, not too deep.

I swim and swim and Uncle sniffs and smiles and when I'm done, he shakes my hand.

"Good job, man," he says. "Your father will love it."

"I hope so. I'm sorry everyone is so sad because of Aunt Diana."

"Aunt Diana? She's not your auntie. She's a very bad lady. She's—she was—my old mother. She threw me away."

"Nicky's sister," I correct him. "She said so."

His mouth freezes open and he stops breathing. And then he sniffs the bottle again very deep.

"That's very complicated," he sighs at last. "My mother and my sister-in-law. It doesn't work for me. I'm throwing Diana away. Nim is handling everything."

†

## MACK

Sean doesn't have a hard time finding Diana hanging out down at the Point with Billy and his new hot wheels. He delivers the letter and the beach cottage key along with an invitation to meet with me on Saturday morning in my office.

I specify that I want her to meet Steven and I alone, with Sean as her personal escort. I think about inviting our lawyer but in the end, dismiss it. We're not down to that yet. I also ask Sunny to join us as my executive assistant.

Steven, Sunny and I know more about Diana than we ever wanted to know, but Sean and Diana are conveniently clueless about the situation. Steven arranges for Prince to serve a formal business breakfast of coffee and pastries and he performs flawlessly, dressed impeccably in his chef's gear.

Diana is a stunning but disturbing woman. After introductions, she's constantly distracted, leering at Prince and Steven both as if she's trying to decide on an entrée. Prince pours the coffee and then goes back to the kitchen for the pastry tray.

"Diana Dixon," I start, "I'm pleased to meet you, but unfortunately you have me confused with my father. I'm only 36 years old. Dr. David Mack, Sr. has been dead for fifteen years. I assume your letter was intended for him, not me.

"I really don't think I can help you. What's done is water under the bridge. Your letter says that you gave your child away when he was six. I don't see any obligation on our part, even if Dad was the father.

"So what is it you want?"

She has no answer except 'money' and even she can't stomach putting it that bluntly. She crosses her long legs and points the toes of her boots, trying to find some leverage in her body.

"I named my son David after him," she says finally. "He promised to support him. I just want what he promised."

"And where is your son now? How does any money we give you support him?"

It's cut and dried. She hasn't got a leg to stand on. She turns her attention to Steven and turns on the charm like a faucet.

"You married?" she purrs. He nods. "Kids?" And now he shows her all his teeth.

"Hundreds," he exaggerates.

"Of course. You look just like him. He was an irresistible rake. How about the boys you were with last week? Is your brother available now?"

"Leave him alone, Diana," he warns. "He's sick. And my son is a little too young for you. What happened to Billy? He was my best friend."

"Billy's hot," she grins. "But he's very expensive. I don't see how I can afford to keep him much longer."

Prince returns to the room with a beautiful silver tray filled with Danish pastries and the conversation shifts. For the first time, I see my brother turn on the seduction and he's a master. He puts one finger on his lips to teasingly hide his smile.

"You're much more beautiful than your sister," he purrs. "Before she left she told me you might be staying at her beach cottage. We had an arrangement."

He winks at her and she nearly falls out of her chair.

"Uh, what kind of arrangement?" she stammers.

"It would be different for you," he mulls. "Free rent at the beach pad. Take care of Billy, but no drugs. How much do you need?"

"Seventy-five hundred," she smiles greedily.

"Shit. You're easy," he laughs.

"A month."

"Mmm. No way. $4K max. If you need more, you can pimp Billy. He's very industrious."

Prince drops the serving tray with a loud clatter on the table and a few of the pastries slide off onto the bare wood.

"Sorry, sorry!" he mumbles visibly distraught as he quickly gathers up the errant Danishes and wraps them in a napkin. After all, we put our dirty bare feet up on the table.

As he hurries from the room to dispose of the escaped pastries, Diana admires his rear view with a growl.

"Nice looking young man. I was even younger when I met your father."

"So that makes you old enough to be his mother," Sim scolds protectively. "Lay off the kids, Diana."

"And how about you?" she smiles suggestively. "What do want in exchange?"

"Nada. Nothing. I'm married to the most beautiful woman on the planet. Don't come around here anymore. Don't hassle my family. If you need anything, talk to Sean. If I find out that any of the money goes to drugs, we're done. Is that a deal?"

She considers her options, but gets off the couch and reluctantly shakes his hand just as Prince returns to the office.

"I wish—" she starts.

"In your fucking wildest dreams," he snorts as he shows her to the door with his patented lady-killer smile. "Thanks, man," he tells Sean. Too easy. Way too easy to be true, I think.

†

S&M

Man, I've got the Universe tied up like a little ball of string in the pocket of my leather pants.

Once the bitch leaves, I go home and tap on my own front door timidly. I don't want to interrupt anything.

Nicky opens the door with a pout on her lips and hugs me.

"Done?" she asks.

"We are so clean, we squeek," I laugh. "I don't think we'll see Diana again. You, uh, okay?"

"*I'm* fine," she groans, "but Kama Dave isn't playing. He won't even dance. What's wrong with him? He's just sitting out on the deck sniffing the stupid oil."

"Poor little sister," I groan. "Do you want me to dance for you?"

I feel good. I bump my hips slowly from side to side and bite my bottom lip. That turns all her lights back on and she winces with pleasure.

"Why didn't you tell me how hot your sister is?" I tease. "You like to play rough, but she's the real deal. She's as rough as it comes. Runs in the family?"

She opens her mouth to scold me but her heart isn't in it. Instead she looks in my eyes and I can see all the soft sweetness hiding behind her act.

"Go home, Nicky," I say. "Let me talk to baby Dave and fix everything, okay?"

Dave is spacing out on the futon on the yoga deck. He starts a little when he sees me and his eyes widen, but he doesn't say a word.

"Talk to me, man," I scold him gently. "What the fuck is up now?"

He goes back to inspecting the forest tree tops and ignores me. I put my hand on his shoulder and lower my voice.

"She's gone, baby. She won't be back. She doesn't even know who you are. What part of Divine Perfection is missing here?"

He doesn't answer so I punch him pretty hard. He turns his head and glares at me defiantly and then just turns away again.

"Alright, you're asking for it," I hiss, grabbing his arm and trying to pull him up to his feet for a good fistfight. But he pushes my hands off with an unexpected strength and fairly screams at me: "Nicky's sister!"

"Oooh, what?" I feign innocence. "What?"

"My mother is Nicky's sister," he snarls. "This is very bad, I think."

"Who—?"

"Jack told me. He heard it all. I can't understand how this even happens. How can I marry my mother's sister? Is that even legal?"

"Uh, I don't think so, buddy. But neither is heroin and you liked that very much."

He thinks about it and grimaces and then he starts to swear slowly and methodically.

"Shit. Shit. Motherfuck. I waited six years for her and all the time she was my—auntie. Motherfucking son of a bitch. I can't play with her anymore, Nim. I'm going to prison if I do.

"Is incest a felony or a misdemeanor?" he cries.

"Fuck if I know," I swear, but I'm doing the math and I realize if Dave's marriage isn't legal, then Nicky isn't my sister-in-law and at least *I'm* off the hook for incest. Somehow I don't get a lot of satisfaction out of that.

"Look, Kamadev," I try to soothe him. "Nobody's going to prison. No one can prove anything. You're the only one who recognized her. If you just shut up about it, you're fine."

"DNA tests," he moans.

"I'm you're guardian. No one can make you take a test and no one's asking for one. Nicky doesn't know anything. Diana doesn't know either.

"Shit," I laugh. "Do you know your mother was asking if you're available? Now *that* would be very bad, man. But you love Nicky. Don't hurt her. Don't tell her."

"I don't know, Nim. I don't know!" he whines. "I'm on probation. What am I supposed to do?"

"What *I* do when I'm in trouble," I offer, "is talk to Mack. He knows everything. I mean he knows about Diana but he also knows *everything* about compassion and integrity. He says kindness can be more important than truth. Come on."

He gets up to his feet and follows me over to the big house where Mack is still sitting in his study. There's leftover coffee and pastries on the desk and he seems very happy to see us.

"How can I help, brothers?" he smiles kindly.

"Um, Dave was just wondering—is it a misdemeanor or a felony? You know what—incest," I grovel.

"Oh," he laughs. "He knows?" Dave nods, visibly disturbed.

"I actually checked it out with my lawyer, Dave," he reassures him. "It's considered a victimless crime. Shit like this happens all the time when there's confusion about consanguinity, especially with foster kids. I can't begin to imagine the mess Steven's kids are going to step in.

"But in your case, hell, it's perfectly legal in Belgium to marry your aunt. You're certainly not going to get arrested if that's what you're worried about."

He pushes the tray of pastries towards Dave and smiles. "We've got your back, brother."

"See? I told you," I snort. "Mack was my teacher. You can always ask him if you don't believe me."

Mack laughs. "Mr. Equanimity. How is *your* wife?"

"Much better, thank you," I grovel some more. "I've been working on that—very hard."

"It's a full time job," he winks. "Don't ever quit. I'll tell you though, whoever came up with the marriage vows must have known something about yoga, about union. 'For better or for worse' is straight out of the practice of Vairagia, dispassion.'"

"Not being attached to your fears or your desires," Dave recites.

"Good. Right," Mack smiles. "Being able to experience both the things you don't want and what you do, coming and going, without getting all tangled up in them. And that, baby brother, is freedom, liberation. Don't let it get complicated, Dave. Don't beat yourself up over it."

Finally, finally! I see some of Dave's teeth emerge behind his tight lips.

"Don't beat myself up," he grins. "That's the best advice I've ever heard. Nicky is much better at it."

†

NAT

Rick, Nick and I are working out in the gym by the pool. I'm still doing moderate basic rehab on my back, Rick is pumping himself into divine perfection and Nick is throwing herself into the weights like a madwoman.

For a moment I think she might burst a vein but she stops suddenly and goes over to the edge of mats and tosses her breakfast onto the lawn.

"Sorry. Sorry," she whines. "I don't feel well."

"Don't go so hard," Rick advises. "Sometimes less is better."

"Yeah, enough," I agree. "Time out."

We crash on the lawn sofa and sit back to watch Rick finish off his delts and arms. It's the best show on Earth.

"You okay?" I ask Nicky.

"Fine," she groans. "Perfection. But that shit Sunny taught me doesn't work. I've been taking my basal temperature every day for two weeks and it's always the same. 99.4. How can I chart my temperature if it's the same every day? Pretty useless I think. Why bother?"

I sit on that for about two minutes and wonder how to tell her. A constant elevated temperature is one of the earliest indicators. She's pregnant.

"Nicky," I suggest, "maybe Kama Dave hasn't got the conservation of his seminal fluids perfected. How can you be sure? I mean with dream sex, what's real and what's a dream? I'm just saying—"

She looks at me curiously and then I see all the lights come on at once. "You don't think?" she gasps.

"Oh, no. No, impossible," she repeats. "He's very careful. He's fucking impeccable."

"Nothing's impossible, sweetheart. But I'll bet he'll be a wonderful father. Look how beautiful Sim's son is."

Sim and Dave are walking across the lawn towards us with Jack nearly dancing with joy behind them, happy to have their attention again. Before anyone has a chance to say a word, Nicky stands up and pushes her first finger hard into Sim's chest.

"Steven Mack," she hisses, "I need to have a word with you in private."

†

## NICK

He winces at the sound of his name. I know he doesn't like it much, but it opens his ears so he can hear what's coming next.

He puts his arm around my waist as we walk back to the Ice House but I pull it off me. I'm furious but I'm not sure whose fault this is. It was Dave's idea but I encouraged him. And S&M can't be blamed because we took advantage of him when he was disturbed.

It's not pregnancy that's worrying me now; it's paternity. Who the fuck is the father? Dave's very controlled, but S&M has been all over the map. I don't speak to him until we get to Mack's office and I calmly ask if we can have some privacy to talk.

The two brothers exchange some worried glances, but Mack is happy to let us use the office and shuts the door as he leaves.

It's all my fault. It was my choice and I liked it a lot. I can't blame him, but I have to know.

"What did you do, S&M?" I accuse him. "What were you thinking?"

"Look, Nick," he apologizes. "I really didn't know she was his mother until now. I was just trying to protect you. It's not really as bad as you think. It's perfectly legal in some countries."

"What?" I'm really confused by that. "What's legal?"

He stops cold. "What are we talking about?" he continues as smooth as silk.

"I'm pregnant, baby," I groan. "But I don't know if it's Dave. I don't know what to think."

"Oh," he reflects. "Oh, that."

"When we—I mean when you—weren't you being safe?"

"Fuck, Nick," he sneers. "I was completely out of control. You ravaged me. Dream sex, shit! You nearly killed me, woman."

"So?"

"So, yes. I dreamed I was pouring milk and honey all over the top of the mountain. I dreamed I filled the whole pond up with milk. I don't think there was an ounce of safe left in me. I warned you, baby."

He sounds serious but his eyes are filled with light and he's got one hand covering he's mouth like he's trying to control his joy.

"It could be Dave," he observes. "I seem to remember he wasn't showing much restraint either that night. It could very possibly be Dave."

He picks a corner off one of the leftover pastries and chews on it while he pours himself some cold coffee.

"Does it really matter, Nick?" he smirks. "I know you love me, baby. I can be the Godfather anyway. At least we're sure the baby is yours!"

†

## PRINCE ALBERT

In the morning I serve breakfast for a business meeting in Dr. Mack's study. It's just coffee and pastries, which doesn't give me much chance to be creative, but I dress in my best chef clothing and comb my hair very nice and neat.

Officer Sean shows up with a mean and twisted looking woman with a very heavy narcotics vibe. She makes me extremely nervous and keeps staring at me at the same time as she's flirting with the boss. I get so disturbed I nearly pour the coffee all over her.

But then it gets worse. I try not to listen to the conversation but he starts smiling very suggestively at her and offers to pay her rent and give her money. From what I hear it sounds like he just bought another girlfriend.

I can understand if a man is married, but I was pretty confused that he could have a girlfriend, too. It really bothered me when he locked his wife up for a week and was fooling around with Nicky and Dave, but this shit takes the cake!

Why would he want to keep yet another woman, a mean wicked woman? He made a deal with her in front of his brother! How can he make love to five people? How many more are there? Where do I stand in all this? He asked me to marry him and he wasn't just teasing, he was cruel. My ears start burning. He's teasing everyone and lying.

The second he leaves the room, I leave all the service on the table and go home. I leave the pastries and the coffee and the plates and swear I'll never serve him again. I go back to my room and there are the cookbooks he gave me, the clothes he bought me, and everything I own but I don't even have a suitcase to pack them in.

I check my phone and see 26 missed messages. Cat is after me and I don't want to play with her any more. I remember him down on his knees in front of everyone, pretending he wanted me, secretly laughing at me. I remember him teaching me how to breathe. I thought he loved me and I trusted him and I even put my hand on his heart.

I've got some money and I can leave, but there's no place for me now. There's a little stash of Cabernet Sauvignon under my bed I was saving for his dinner. It's a very nice vintage and I pull one of the corks out and drink straight off the bottleneck.

That makes me feel a little better but I want to hurt him very badly. I want him to know how much I hurt. I've still got my gun but there's nothing but blanks in it.

I put my headset on and listen to Five Finger Death Punch, 'Just Walk Away', as loud as it can get. I'm starting to feel very mellow and mad at the same time. By the time I open the second bottle, I've got it all figured out.

†

## S&M

"New rules," I purr. "No more wild card snake-eye double Shiva immunity. Just for tonight, okay? I've had enough madness for one day. I blame the fool moon for everything."

"Full moon," Nicky corrects me.

"No kidding," I snort.

I toss the dice on the boardroom table and get a 3 and a 5, hard to beat without the wild card rule. Dave rolls a 1 and a 3 to tie me. Nicky rolls a pair of 3's and loses.

"Sick rules, S&M," she snorts. "It's twisted."

"You can't win, Nicky," Dave teases. "But you can't quit. Not until we win all of your—um, whatdya got tonight?"

She gives him a piercing look and takes the dice prisoner in her hands, stopping the game. "A lot more than you think, Kama Dave, sir. You're not my only baby now, sugar."

She sets the dice back on the table and puts both her hands on her belly with that Mona Lisa smile and watches his face carefully. He's not even breathing.

He just sits there watching her without a trace of emotion. So I punch him. He looks over at me in a daze and wonders. "Mine?"

I shrug my shoulders. "I sure hope so."

Then he looks at her and asks again, "Mine?" and she just shrugs. "Uh," he grunts. "I thought dream sex was a pretty good invention."

Then he runs a hand through his hair as if he's checking to see if he needs a haircut, grabs a fistful of it and pulls hard.

"Fuck, we're pregnant?"

I'm waiting for him to start crying in confusion but he howls with joy instead. "It fucking must have worked," he laughs. And then he shows her his canine teeth and growls, "I'm not a baby."

Well and good. He's taking it very nicely. I let out a sigh of relief. I'm hungry as shit all of a sudden. Brandy comes in through the kitchen and Dave jumps up and hugs her.

"Mom!" he laughs, "You're going to be a grandmother!"

My wife is either going to be an adopted grandmother, an auntie or, I think, possibly the stepmother of another one of my bastards. I feel so light-headed I have to put my face down on the table to catch my breath. I haven't eaten anything but some pastry crumbs and coffee all day.

I'm ravenous. Since when does the chef take Saturday night off? There's nothing cooking in the kitchen so I knock on his bedroom door. When he doesn't answer, I figure he's got his music blaring so I open the door and peek in.

He's lying on the bed with his headset on but when I shake him, he's stiff and cold. There's two empty wine bottles on the table, a bottle of Z's and a piece of paper with a note.

*Steven, I love you but I don't know how. P.*

I scream for Brandy, then put my mouth on his cold lips and try to teach him how to breathe.

†

## PRINCE ALBERT

My stomach hurts. My chest aches and my throat hurts; my head is banging and I try to find some place in my body where there's no pain. My feet don't hurt but I feel my toes cramping and twitching.

"Awwww," I moan. "Fuck." Then I open my eyes and I feel the most horrible pain of all, like a knife twisting right in the middle of my heart.

He's sitting in the chair next to my bed watching me with those ice blue eyes. He cuts my heart open with his stare and sends a chill through me. I'm so cold. I have an IV needle in my arm and I'm covered with blankets but I'm still shivering.

"Don't ever do that to me again," he says quietly, but his voice doesn't match his eyes. His voice is low and kind and a little bit shaky.

"I'm supposed to let Dr. Jain know when you wake up, but I'd like to talk to you first. Is that okay?"

I nod but then he holds up the little note I wrote and I shake my head hard. I don't want to talk about that. I'd rather be dead. I meant to be dead.

"'*Steven*'," he reads. "Steven? Man, you really know how to hurt a guy."

"It's your name!" I croak. Aw, my esophagus burns on the words. If he reads the rest of it out loud, I will show him hurt! I've got my knives and I can get bullets on the Internet! I close my eyes in pain and wait for the rest.

I wait as if hearing him read the note to me is a death sentence. When he doesn't go on, I open my eyes and watch him fold the note and stuff it into his pocket. He's done reading. Instead, he looks seriously at me.

"I love you, too. I haven't always loved you," he laughs. "I wanted to kill you when I met you. But I love you very much now. And I'm definitely not gay."

"How would you know?" I ask him suspiciously.

"Give me a minute," he sighs and he leaves the room and comes back a few minutes later with two cups.

"You sound like shit. They had to pump your stomach out. Nat made this for your throat. Calendula and rose tea with lavender honey. Try it."

It tastes sweet and nourishing and I start to relax a little. He leans back in the chair and puts his big bare feet up on my bed. I give him a dirty look but he sighs and looks at me pathetically.

"Do you really mind? I mean, I've been sitting here since yesterday babysitting you and I'm very tired."

He drops his head back and watches the ceiling for a little bit and then I see his eyes close. I think he may have fallen asleep and I wonder if he's going to drop the cup of tea in his hand.

I watch him and wait. He looks very tired and sad but he hasn't answered.

"How would you know?" I ask again.

"I'm not wired that way," he finally says without opening his eyes. "I mean sexually, physically and energetically it doesn't work for me.

"The rest of it, on the emotional, mental and spiritual levels, I'm a yogi slut. I love everybody. 'A yogi's love is like the sun: it shines on everyone.'

"But my body—my circuits—only work with women. I'm just not attracted the other way."

He picks his head up and finishes off the tea. "I'm pretty sure you're not gay either," he smiles. "But you were right about one thing. You don't know what love is. You haven't got a clue."

He swings his feet off the bed, leans over and puts his hand on my arm, right on the IV.

"Man, you caused a lot of drama last night and you missed the whole show. Dr. Jain has to check you out now and I'm pretty sure with a suicide attempt he's required by law to refer you to a psychiatrist.

"But I'll come back when he's done talking to you, okay?"

"Thank you," I mumble. My throat feels better. "I'm sorry, man."

"Just between you and me," he adds, "*you* can call me 'Steven'. But not in front of anyone. It will just be a private understanding between us, Prince." And then he adds with a wink, "Honey."

†

NAT

Every one of us is shocked and disturbed by the trauma but I feel especially culpable. Sim warned me a few days ago that he was concerned about Prince and I naively assumed a massage fixed everything. Looking back, I wonder that we didn't worry more.

Sure, he's a disturbed teenager, but considering he was out on the street dealing drugs when he was twelve, he's been putting on a pretty slick act. He had money, freedom, talent, creativity and the respect of everyone in the house but—unless he was shopping or working in the kitchen—he rarely left his room.

Nothing seemed out of the ordinary last night. If Sim hadn't been so hungry, Prince would be dead.

After the ambulance leaves, after the EMTs pump his stomach, after Brandy cleans up the vomit, gives him a bed bath and tucks him in with an IV and a kiss, Sim sits with him in a suicide watch. Rick comes to bed exhausted and cries.

Prince is still unconscious in the morning, so I channel my distress in the lab. Dave and I blend herb teas and abhyanga oils targeted for detoxification and emotional balance. The 'Rx Prince' blend Dave concocted is brilliant so we mix up a bigger batch.

There's no such thing as an instant fix, I remind myself. I should have followed up. Dave watches me sulking over the herbs and oils and puts an arm around me.

"Don't beat yourself up, Nat," he smiles. "It's very good advice."

Rick is waiting in the boardroom and I sit with him while Dave makes tea.

"Legally and ethically, I'm required to report a suicide attempt and refer him to psychiatric help," he says. "I don't feel right about shipping him to the hospital, Nat. He's a minor and a runaway and I don't want to see him end up as a ward of the state.

"I think you and Sim can handle it, but I have to be sure. If I'm wrong and he does it again, well, it'll be fucked if I'm wrong."

I'm not a psychiatrist but both Sim and I are certified yoga therapists. I think we've got a good shot at it. We've done a good job with Dave, I think, as he serves us a taste of the medicinal tea. He could have just as easily been committed to a prison or institutionalized.

Then I realize we're all institutionalized here; it's just a very weird institution—medical, spiritual, sexual and mental. We've created our own blend of retreat, rehabilitation center, infirmary, orphanage, casino and strip club.

"Prince Charming is awake," Sim jokes half-heartedly as he comes out of the bedroom. "Oooh, the tea smells magic. Can I have five minutes before you check on him, Jain?" he requests pouring a couple cups. "Thanks." And he disappears again.

"We can do it, Rick," I promise. "We love him."

"Let me be the judge of that," he sighs. "Let me see what he has to say for himself."

†

JAIN

"I know it hurts to talk," I tell him while I check his pulse and blood pressure, "so don't try to explain, buddy, but I need to ask a few questions.

"Sim says you left him a note. I haven't seen it, but he thinks you did this on purpose. It doesn't look like you were just trying to get stoned. Is he right?"

He winces but nods.

"Okay then, I'm required to get you some psychiatric help. There's already a medical report since we had to get the EMTs up here. You haven't got a guardian and I'm afraid if I send you to the hospital it's going to be a one-way trip for you.

"You put me in a really bad spot. Hell, don't look at me like that, I'm trying to help."

His eyes are wide with horror and he's shaking his head in disbelief.

"Nah," he croaks, "I was just mad. I won't do it again."

"Okay then, let me help. Why were you mad?"

"Ask him," he sneers.

"Sim? Are you still mad at him?"

"I don't know," he moans. "I don't know. I don't think so."

"I want to keep you here," I explain. "Nat and Sim could help if you let them, but if you're mad at Sim that might be a problem."

"I'll let them," he begs. "Whatever. Please, Doc."

"I'll talk to Mack. If we both recommend therapy instead of a psychiatric evaluation, we might be able to do this. But you have to work with us. Man, why didn't you talk to someone?"

"I just wanted to go. But I was afraid to."

"Afraid to be back on the street?" It's a pretty easy guess. I don't want to traumatize him any further. He looks horribly agitated.

"Okay. I want you to sleep some more. Nat will bring you some more herbs and maybe do some massage and Sim will sit with you. We can't leave you alone for a while.

"Maybe we'll have to move you to IC and put the nurses on watch, but let's see how you go. Can you sleep?"

"Mmm," he nods.

I open the door and wave Nat and Sim in. Nat brings more tea and then goes back, returning with clean towels, oil and fresh cut flowers. Prince smiles at her gratefully.

"I want him to sleep," I instruct them. "I'll leave him in your hands and we can talk about therapy later. If you need me, I'll be in Mack's office dealing with the paperwork.

"Oh," I remember. "He said to ask you, Sim. What was in the note? Why was he so mad?"

Sim eases back into the chair with a tired smile. "Ah, it's pretty simple, Jain," he explains. "A teenage identity crisis. I can guarantee it won't happen again."

†

## S&M

"So?" I wonder, "What did he say?"

"Work with you or go to the psycho ward," he sniffs. "I don't want to go."

"Good, boy," I give him an evil laugh. "You're at our mercy now."

He tries to smile but he looks nervous. We still haven't cracked his ice. Nat pulls back the bottom of the covers to expose his feet and he groans.

"I'm fucking freezing," he objects.

"Not for long," she promises. "I want to help you sleep. We'll do longer massages later but for now I'm only going to do your feet. We've mixed up some very powerful stuff and the feet are a great vehicle for sleep aids."

She starts rubbing his feet with the sweet smelling oils and I can nearly taste the sharp citrus of the bergamot in the air, with holy basil and laurel undertones.

"Ah, me too, baby," I groan. "I'm beaten to death. I need to sleep, too. I'm next."

"Sure, boss," she purrs. "I'll do your feet, too."

"The first rule, Prince," I scold him, "is you can't wear shoes any more. You'll be a lot more grounded with bare feet."

"I can't work in a kitchen without shoes," he complains.

"You won't be cooking for a while. Trust me. No shoes."

"Who's going to cook?" he frets.

"Me. Sunny. Nat. Dave. We're all great cooks. We never really needed a chef. We just wanted you to stay."

He looks offended but then I see the lights coming on, one by one. *We didn't need you. We wanted you.* He's never had parents who cared for him. He doesn't know what love is, even when it smacks him in the face.

"Move over, honey," I growl. "I need to sleep, too."

"What? No! Not with me. Fuck off, Steven," he snorts indignantly and Nat suppresses a laugh.

"Don't make me handcuff you to the bed, man," I threaten. "I need my foot massage. If I can't get some sleep here, I'm going to be very pissed."

"Move over, Prince," Nat assures him. "He's slept with Dr. Jain. He's slept with me. He'll sleep with anybody. Think of him as a big dog. You're very safe."

I give him a shove rough enough to nearly pull the IV out. He scoots over and I lie down next to him with a big gratified sigh.

"Ahhhh. Man! Do you feel that?"

"What?"

"Can't you feel it? It's incredible!"

"What? What?" he's annoyed as hell.

"The incredible—irresistible—electric charge, the electromagnetic kundalini attraction! You can't feel it?"

"What the fuck are you talking about?" he moans.

"Yeah. I thought so," I laugh. "I don't feel it either. I don't feel a thing. I'm just not—attracted to you, honey. Sorry."

"You're making fun of me," he groans.

"Yeah. Relax. I wouldn't abuse you if you paid me. Remember what you said? *'You can't afford me'*? That was pretty amusing. I actually can. Tell him, Nat."

"We're both yoga therapists, baby," she explains. "We have to carry personal liability insurance. What've you got, Sim? A couple million?"

"Four million. I would be amazed if I could cause four million dollars in personal injuries by teaching yoga, but that's standard coverage."

"Yeah, me too. It's amusing," she agrees. "So, Prince, you know how doctors have to carry malpractice insurance? In addition to liability and medical coverage, yoga teachers and therapists are insured for sexual misconduct and assault.

"If he misbehaves, you can sue him for a cool four million and he's covered."

"Two million for each occurrence," I correct her, "I'd have to harass both of you at once for the full coverage.

"Nat, do you think it would be considered assault or sexual misconduct if I accidentally caused someone to have a spontaneous orgasm?" I tease.

"Nah," she plays along with me. "Orgasms come from the inside out. If he gets off from hearing you snore, I don't think you can be held accountable."

"Then you're safe with me, honey," I assure him. "Sweet dreams. Breathe, damn it!"

I can see his teeth and a little grin breaking through as the ice starts to melt. Nat tucks his feet in and starts on mine. I feel the bergamot, laurel and tulsi penetrating my skin and dissolving into all the nerve endings in the soles of my feet.

"There was something Nat said," I sigh. "'When you can look pain in the eye—when you submit—you open the doorway to becoming a great being.'

"Yes, yes, Nat baby," I hum. "I think we'll keep you. I think we'll keep Prince too." I close my eyes and see the fireworks of fatigued brain cells and optic nerves giving up the ghost. "Yes."

All the lights are turning on, and I feel the colors creeping up my spine: red, orange, yellow, green, blue, indigo and violet, mixing at the top of my head in a pure white light.

I hear Prince exhale a long breath as he quits struggling against the Universe.

"Sweet dreams, Steven," he sighs and his next inhale breaks with a little Ujjayi snort.

I disappear in underwater dreams listening to the soundtrack of his soft snores.

## EPILOGUE

*"The hunger for love is much more difficult to remove than the hunger for bread."* ~ Mother Teresa

†

MACK

Jack Mack doesn't sleep in the Nurses' room anymore. The ladies call it the Nursery now and their new passion is remodeling it. Even though Nicky isn't showing yet, she's expecting twins.

The ultrasound revealed two boys, but they're fraternal, not identical twins. Fraternal twins are conceived with two separate eggs by two separate sperm. Nicky fainted with joy when she got the news.

Kama Dave doesn't cry anymore.

Jack sleeps out on the deck of the pool house now, an incorrigible nature boy like his father. He's negotiated a deal with Brandy: Fang can visit him on the deck but not in the house.

Prince is back in the kitchen again but he's a changed man since the suicide attempt. He ordered wall-to-wall mats for the kitchen and no longer wears shoes or a shirt, even when he's serving the meal. For a while, he donned shoes to go shopping but somehow he's managed to get around that, too. I suspect it has something to do with his huge expense account at the markets.

None of the women are complaining about having another piece of eye candy wandering around the premises. When he's not working, he's lifting weights, swimming, sun bathing and exploring the forest, no longer hiding in his room listening to heavy metal.

If you get up early enough in the morning, before dawn, you can see the new Sunrise ritual as Kama Dave and Prince Albert come out of the Fire House barefoot and shirtless in the dark on their way to their yoga lesson. An hour and a half later, they head home with Jack in tow for breakfast.

Steven spends the dawn hour teaching them asana, pranayama and meditation, but when the class is over, he goes back to bed for his personal Sadhana, his favorite Tantric yoga practice: teaching his wife how to make the Universe spin.

†††

## † YOGA SANSKRIT APPENDIX †

**Abhyanga** – Ayurvedic massage
**Asana** – Physical yoga postures
**Kosha** – One of the five layers of consciousness ranging from the gross physical layer to the most subtle spiritual level. (House of Pain, pp. 22 – 23)
**Maya** – The illusion of duality in the phenomenal universe
**Mudra** – Ritual hand movements and gestures used to indicate an idea or promote a specific flow of energy to improve concentration, comprehension and memory.
**Nadi Shodana** – Alternate nostril breathing to create pranic balance
**Nirvana** – The word literally means "blown out" (as in a candle) and refers, in the Buddhist context, to the imperturbable stillness of mind after the fires of desire, aversion, and delusion have been finally extinguished.
**Prana (n) Pranic (adj)** – Life force energy (also Qi or Chi). Prana is regulated by the neuroendocrine system and can be influenced by breath, postures and concentration.
**Pranayama** – Controlled breathing techniques.
**Sattvic** – Having the quality of purity, perfection and flawlessness.
**Sadhana** – An individual's yoga practice or path
**Tantra** – An esoteric branch of yoga embracing sensory pleasures as tools for enlightenment.
**Tantrika** – A female Tantric practitioner.
**Ujjayi** – A pranayama to slow the breath by restricting the glottis in the throat, similar to a snore.
**Vairagya** – Dispassion, equanimity, one of the highest goals of yoga; freedom from attachment to both desires and aversions.

www.ingramcontent.com/pod-product-compliance
Lightning Source LLC
Chambersburg PA
CBHW051233260626
47162CB00002B/408

*9780615814803*